GET FIT NOW FOR

# HIGH SCHOOL
# BASKETBALL

GET FIT NOW FOR

# HIGH SCHOOL
# BASKETBALL

## THE COMPLETE GUIDE FOR ULTIMATE PERFORMANCE

### JOSEPH KOLB

PHOTOGRAPHY BY
**PETER FIELD PECK**

A GETFITNOW.COM BOOK
Hatherleigh Press CPL YA
New York • London

GetFitNow.com Books
Hatherleigh Press
5-22 46th Avenue, Suite 200
Long Island City, NY 11101
**www.GetFitNow.com**

Library of Congress Cataloging-in-Publication Data

Kolb, Joseph J.
Get fit now for high school basketball / Joseph J. Kolb.
    p. cm.
 Includes bibliographical references.
ISBN 1-57826-094-9 (paper : alk. paper)
1.  Basketball for children–Training–Handbooks, manuals, etc.–Juvenile literature. [1. Basketball–Training.]  I. Title.
GV886.25.K65 2002
796.323'07'7–dc21

                                                2002068942


Cover design by Angel Harleycat
Interior design by Tai Blanche


Printed in Canada
10  9  8  7  6  5  4  3  2  1

# Table of Contents

Acknowledgements . . . . . . . . . . . . . . . . . . . . . . .6

Dedication . . . . . . . . . . . . . . . . . . . . . . . . . . . .7

1 Conditioning the High School Athlete . . . . . .9

2 Step 1: Performance Evaluation . . . . . . . . .15

3 Principles of Basketball Nutrition . . . . . . . .40

4 Flexibility Training . . . . . . . . . . . . . . . . . . .52

5 Coordination and Agility Training . . . . . . . .75

6 Principles of Strength Training . . . . . . . . . .89

7 Principles of Endurance Training . . . . . . . .121

8 Speed Training . . . . . . . . . . . . . . . . . . . . .125

9 Power Training . . . . . . . . . . . . . . . . . . . . .137

10 Vision Training . . . . . . . . . . . . . . . . . . . . .151

11 Mental Training . . . . . . . . . . . . . . . . . . . .156

12 Overtraining . . . . . . . . . . . . . . . . . . . . . . .160

13 Game Day . . . . . . . . . . . . . . . . . . . . . . . .164

14 Injury Reconditioning . . . . . . . . . . . . . . . .168

15 No Shortcuts . . . . . . . . . . . . . . . . . . . . . .226

16 The Female Player . . . . . . . . . . . . . . . . . .233

17 Wheelchair Basketball . . . . . . . . . . . . . . .238

18 Six-Month Training Program . . . . . . . . . . .251

# Acknowledgements

After over 20 years in athletic training I've had the opportunity to experience much of what the field has to offer. The ability to do this was supported by my family, to whom I am greatly indebted. My family, like many others in this field, have had to make sacrifices in social and even family occasions and personal availability. I thank God for their love and understanding through the years and for making it easy for me to achieve my goals and participate in events which may have taken time away from us.

To my wife Rachael, my daughters Jessica, Christina and JoAnne and my son John, thank you. I am indebted to my parents Ann and John who gave me the foundation and tools to embark upon a career as a dedicated professional and parent.

Special thanks go to my editor Lori Baird and Kevin Moran, Publisher of Hatherleigh Press, for their confidence and assistance in publishing this book.

I also want to thank the following people for their assistance in this project. Frank Burns, Dan Ferraro, Paul Graves, Charles Harvey, Alyce Kilpatrick, the players and coaches at Christ the King High School and Gallup High School in New Mexico, and John Lomasney.

# Dedication

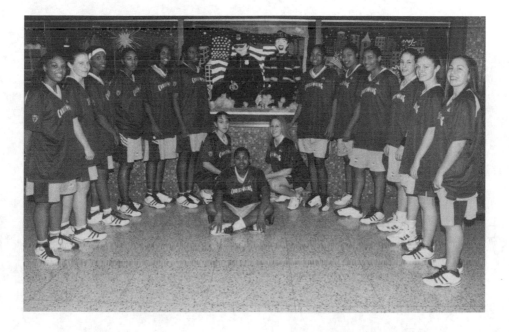

To the heroes and victims of 9/11

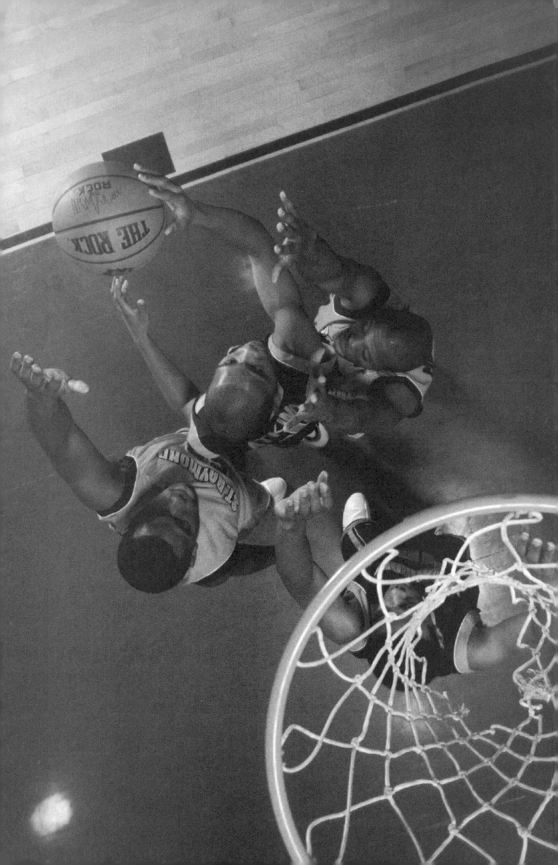

# Chapter 1

# Conditioning the High School Athlete

**F**or decades there has been significant controversy surrounding sport-specific conditioning, especially at the high school level. Those who oppose conditioning argue that high school athletes are too young to engage in rigorous conditioning exercises, that young female athletes risk injury by lifting weights; and that lifting weights will slow the athlete down and affect his or her performance and agility. Experts in the field of strength and conditioning, myself included, know that these arguments are *false, false, false*. Health literature supports the use of conditioning exercises as a valuable, performance-enhancing tool that also prevents injury and aids in the physical and emotional development of the young athlete.

Basketball, like many other high school sports, has evolved into an aggressive contact sport in which only the strong survive and thrive.

It's no accident that all NBA teams and most colleges in the United States employ strength and conditioning coaches or specialists. This sports medicine discipline has dramatically contributed to the "new" basketball player—a stronger, more flexible and well-rounded athlete. Take a look at photos of college and professional basketball players before the 1990s. Without a doubt there were good players; however, many were relying on natural talent to succeed. In today's environment, not only have physiques become more athletic, but baseline to baseline endurance has improved and vertical jump ability has skyrocketed. Today, dribbling through the paint can be like running through a forest of immovable trees.

Let's look at the reasoning behind this remarkable change. There are more than 650 muscles in your body, each of which has the purpose of moving a body segment, whether it's your little toe or a large muscle group, like the quadriceps that move the knee.

You can easily recognize that daily activities require fairly minor force in terms of muscle movement. Now, imagine what force must be produced by your neuromuscular system to dribble a basketball down court and quickly release the ball from the three-point line, all while an opponent is covering you. Or what about performing a lay-up, with the goal of propelling your body through the air as close as possible to the basket? And of course, there's the thrill of it all, slamming the ball down through the rim.

Undoubtedly genetics plays a role in the ability to excel at many of these skills. Equally, developing the body's systems through controlled stresses will increase your ability to do work—and with the right exercises—perform required basketball skills efficiently, competently, and powerfully. This is where sports conditioning can be of enormous use.

The phrase *sports conditioning* may mean lifting weights to you. But if you want to reach new heights (literally and figuratively), lifting weights is only part of the equation. A well-rounded basketball conditioning program will use many different disciplines to improve your overall athletic abilities, including:

- Stretching
- Balance and agility training
- Endurance training
- Nutrition
- Power and speed training
- Strength training
- Vision training

High school coaches have limited time to spend with their athletes and devoting significant time in the weight room on the parameters listed above may seem superfluous, especially if players also need time developing ball-handling skills and game strategies. But balancing all of these activities can—and is—being done with great success. This book will show you how to do just that.

Let's take a moment to explore some of the most common concerns expressed by coaches and parents whose athletes are considering sports conditioning:

## Is It Safe?

Conditioning—weight training especially—is not only safe but also has been found to contribute to the strength of bones, ligaments, and tendons.

## Will the Added Bulk from Weight Training Make Me Slower?

Weight training won't make you slower. *Not* running will make you slower. Strong muscles are needed to propel the body

# GUIDELINES FOR COACHES ON SUCCESSFUL CONDITIONING PROGRAMS

Here are some basic guidelines for coaches to consider when designing a program for their athletes.

Set realistic goals for each player. These can be determined based on pre-season fitness tests.

Use an individualized program for each athlete. Treat your athletes like the individuals they are.

Keep in mind that consistency is key. Lack of consistency is one of the most common mistakes made in high school conditioning programs. Often programs are used just during the pre-season. Jump on board with the program during the pre-season and stick with it to the last day of play. Juggling the parameters of the program can jeopardize its effectiveness. A high school basketball season lasts about three months. If the body isn't stressed—through weight training, for example—not only will strength gains stagnate, they may also diminish. And that will happen toward the end of the season, when you want to be the strongest (hopefully for the playoffs!).

Be mindful of how you use conditioning. Avoid using conditioning as a punishment or applying it haphazardly as something to keep athletes busy before practice now and then.

Develop an award system to motivate the players, and revaluate progress every four to six weeks. Athletes who improve in sport-specific criteria such as vertical jump, baseline to baseline speed, flexibility, bench press, or squat strength should be recognized as a Strong Man or Iron Woman depending on their progress. The coaching staff can develop criteria to recognize players based on the athlete's abilities and team philosophies.

Remember that progress can't be made without occasional overload. The body needs to be safely stressed to increase its abilities.

Attend to the nagging injuries of your athletes. Pain will always get in the way of successful playing and conditioning. Watch your athletes closely. For safety, motivation, and liability purposes, all conditioning sessions need to be supervised by a member of the coaching staff. Teach the athletes how to spot and monitor progress. Athletes and parents must be instructed that additional conditioning at home may accelerate the over-training/burnout syndrome.

Be sure all equipment used in the program is safe and well maintained. This one should be obvious, but it bears repeating.

Vary the program according to the recommendations discussed later in the book. Keep in mind that more is not always better. For instance, the program you follow during the pre-season in the weight room will be different from the program during the season. This concept is called periodization.

Track each session on a chart. Players and managers can manage these.

Maintain a motivating and constructive environment. If training becomes a tedious chore for the coaches, the athletes will assume the same attitude. Approaching conditioning with the same vigor as practicing free throws will provide results that will take your team to new levels of performance.

through space. The stronger the muscles, the greater the force you can exert to move the body. Speed and jumping ability are further enhanced through power drills, which have been proven safe for teenagers.

## How Will It Affect My Appearance?

One of the most common concerns of women considering weight training is the risk that muscle growth will negatively alter their appearance. Using a moderate-intensity sports conditioning program, such as the one included in this book, teenage girls are at no risk of becoming muscle magazine cover girls. For more visible proof, take a look at the women playing basketball at the college and professional level. There's no doubt that women who can dunk a basketball can still have figures like models.

## How Do I Know Which Program to Trust?

One fact about conditioning programs: Everyone's an expert, with a program guaranteed to produce results. It's not unreasonable to survey ten books and magazines and find ten different ways to achieve the same goals. But for high school basketball, time is the one factor that can't be ignored when choosing a program. The programs in this book are all designed with an appreciation of the time constraints imposed on high school coaches. The mentality and logistics of basketball do not allow any athlete to spend five days per week in the weight room. These programs will provide results while minimizing the time off the floor.

# Chapter 2

# Step 1: Performance Evaluation

**G**reat high school basketball players come in all shapes and sizes. While natural basketball skills are obviously important in determining whether a player can be competitive, formally assessing physical capabilities can provide valuable information about what the athlete can do on the court and in which areas the athlete needs to improve, both to enhance performance and prevent injuries. This chapter outlines a simple but effective assessment program designed specifically for basketball athletes.

The adolescent years present unique challenges and opportunities for coaches in terms of predicting an athlete's success. An athlete's capabilities may change from one year to the next because of a growth spurt, or due to changes in physical structure, level of activity or injury. There have been cases in which NBA players were cut from a junior high or high school team only to blossom a year or two later. It's also not uncommon to find an athlete has great basketball skills but deficiencies in some physical fitness aspect that can limit his or her potential.

Evaluating physical fitness allows the coach and athlete to identify any deficits in this area and provide the opportunity for correction. This process also allows the coach to set basketball-specific physical goals unique to the player.

# Evaluating Basketball Physical Fitness

The fundamental parameters of physical fitness are flexibility; coordination and agility; and muscular and cardiorespiratory endurance, strength, and power. The following assessment program is based on a 100-point scale. The athlete scores points based on his or her results. Coaches can use this point system to motivate athletes and monitor the progress of team members.

I recommend including an incentive program based on accumulated points as part of the performance evaluation. Players who accumulate 90 to 100 points receive a T-shirt or certificate or are identified on a bulletin board as the "Iron Player," or another catchy phrase the coach or team agrees upon. Some schools have even recruited their school mascot into the program (the "Iron Bengal," for instance).

A second tier award can be presented to those athletes scoring between 80 and 90 points. A "Most Improved" award should be considered as well. This can motivate high-scoring athletes to improve even further and athletes who didn't score high enough can be recognized for their efforts. The coach will determine the standard, but an improvement of 10 percent, either in individual progress or in total score, is one option.

**Here are some additional points to consider.**

- Evaluations should be conducted three times: at the beginning of the school year, during the pre-season, and in the middle of the season.
- Many of these tests require a stopwatch and tape measure.
- Individual physical fitness charts make it easy to follow and track the athlete's progress. Coaches and athletes can use the following sample evaluation chart to track results.

# SAMPLE INDIVIDUAL PHYSICAL FITNESS CHART

Team Name and Level (e.g., Junior Varsity Girls Basketball)

Athlete's Name:　　　　　　　Grade　　　Position

|  | Test 1 | Test 2 | Test 3 |
|---|---|---|---|
| Date: | | | |
| Height: | | | |
| Weight: | | | |
| Resting Heart Rate: | | | |
| Flexibility: | | | |
| Balance: | | | |
| Agility: | | | |
| Aerobic Fitness: | | | |
| Muscle Endurance: | | | |
| Vertical Jump: | | | |
| Court Speed: | | | |
| Full Court Shuttle: | | | |
| Squat: | | | |
| Bench Press: | | | |
| Total Points: | | | |

**Some important notes:**
- Warm up before the tests; cool down and stretch afterward.
- The tests are best done in stations, by position: guards with guards, forwards with forwards; and with the help of assistants.
- Provide a 5-minute rest between strenuous tests such as the 3/4-court sprint, full court shuttle run, and weights. Lack of recovery can affect validity of results.
- Record any special circumstances that may affect test results. These may include injury and illness.

If the test cannot be completed in one day because of time constraints, you can break the test into two days as follows:

## TWO-DAY FITNESS TESTING PROTOCOL

| Day 1 | Day 2 |
|---|---|
| Resting Heart Rate | Flexibility |
| Height and Weight | Balance Test |
| Agility | Muscle Endurance |
| Aerobic Fitness | Half-Court Speed |
| Full-Court Shuttle | Squats |
| Vertical Jump | Bench Press |

# Physical Fitness Tests

Here is a brief overview of each of the components of the physical fitness test.

## Height and Weight

**PURPOSE:** To identify athletes who are over- or underweight. Weight loss can also indicate dehydration. If an athlete has lost more than 2 percent of their body weight during a workout, he or she needs to rehydrate. A simple rule to remember is that for each pound lost during exercise one pint of liquid should be consumed. Height measurements can identify growth spurts and how they may have affected performance.

**TOOLS:** Ideally, height and weight should be measured with a calibrated medical scale.

**TECHNIQUE:** The athlete should stand on the scale wearing shorts and a T-shirt but no shoes.

## Resting Heart Rate

**PURPOSE:** The resting heart rate is one indicator of cardio-vascular efficiency. The better conditioned the athlete, the lower his or her heart rate will be. An average resting heart rate is between 60 to 80 beats per minute. An increase in resting heart rate can indicate illness, over-training, and/or emotional stress.

**TOOLS:** Watch or stopwatch

**TECHNIQUE:** Have the athlete sit quietly for 10 minutes. This can be done in a classroom while the coach explains the reason and components of the evaluations.

Find the pulse either on the neck (on the side of the throat) or the wrist (on the thumb side between the large tendons in the middle of the wrist and the radius bone). Use the middle three fingers, not the thumb, to measure the pulse.

Count the number of pulses in a 15-second period. Multiply that number by four to calculate resting heart rate for 1 minute. Record the result on the evaluation form.

## Flexibility

**PURPOSE:** To prepare muscles for work and prevent injuries. Lack of, or inadequate stretching, inactivity, or injury can adversely affect flexibility.

**TOOLS:** The sit-and-reach test is a traditional favorite for evaluating hamstring and trunk flexibility. Sit-and-reach boxes are available at most sporting goods stores. Most boxes are 12 inches high. For taller basketball players (who typically have larger feet) fitting into this device can be difficult, so a 14- to 16-inch box may be better.

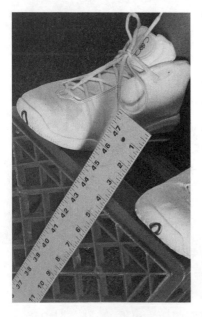

**TECHNIQUE:** Place a ruler on the top edge of the box at the 4-inch mark.

Place the box against the wall with the 12-inch mark of the ruler facing the wall. Have the athlete sit on the floor, with his or her feet placed against the box.

Have the athlete put one hand over the other.

The athlete should take a deep breath and *slowly* move his or her fingers along the ruler. The athlete should not jerk forward or lift the legs off the ground.

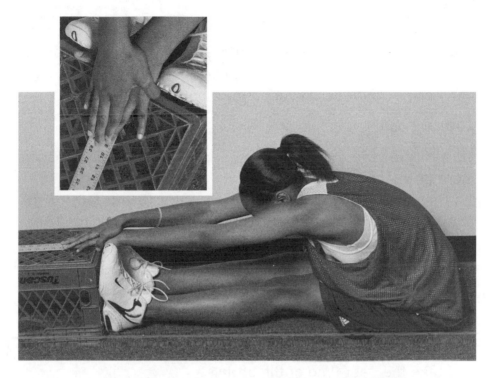

Have the athlete stop at the point of maximum tension, where there is *no* pain. Mark the distance on the ruler. Repeat the test two more times and take the best distance of the three trials.

**SCORING.** Use the following chart to score the flexibility test.

| FLEXIBILITY SCORING CHART | | | |
| --- | --- | --- | --- |
| **Male** | **Points** | **Female** | **Points** |
| 11 inches | 10 | 12 inches | 10 |
| 8 to 10 inches | 8 | 10 to 11 inches | 8 |
| 3 to 7 inches | 6 | 6 to 9 inches | 6 |
| 1 to 2 inches | 4 | 2 to 5 inches | 4 |
| 1 inch | 0 | 2 inches | 0 |

## Balance

**PURPOSE:** This test measures the athlete's ability to control and react to changes in balance. Good balance can help players respond more quickly to plays or potential injuries.

**TOOLS:** None.

**TECHNIQUE:** The stork test is a simple yet effective measurement of the athlete's balance.

The athlete should stand on one leg with the foot of the other leg resting on the inside of the straight leg at the knee, keeping the arms out to the side at shoulder level. Eyes should be closed.

Time how long the athlete can hold the position without losing balance, dropping the foot, or twisting the foot of the straight leg.

Alternate feet after each bout. Repeat process three times and take the best time of three trials.

**SCORING:** Use the same point scale for both male and female players.

| BALANCE SCORING CHART ||
| :--- | :--- |
| **Time** | **Points** |
| 10 sec. and longer | 10 |
| 8 to 10 sec. | 8 |
| 6 to 7 sec. | 6 |
| 4 to 5 sec. | 4 |
| Less than 4 sec. | 0 |

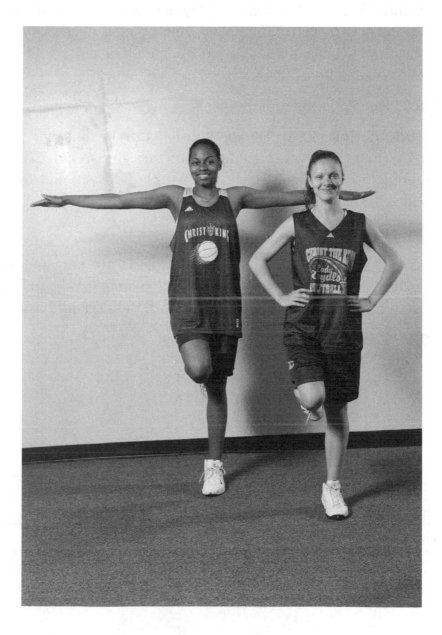

## Agility

**PURPOSE:** Basketball requires agility and quickness. The side-step shuffle is a test that gauges lateral speed necessary for maneuvers such as defending an opponent or cutting to get open for a pass.

**TOOLS:** 2 cones, rope or line

**TECHNIQUE:** The player will side shuffle laterally right and left, keeping knees bent and back and head straight. To move laterally, bring the feet together and then separate them quickly.

Place two cones 10 yards apart. Place a line between the cones at the five-yard point.

Have the player stand over the middle line.

At "go" the player side shuffles back and forth between the cones for 20 seconds, counting each time a cone is tapped. The object is to tap the cone on each end with the nearest hand.

**SCORING.** Use the following charts to score the agility test.

| AGILITY SCORING CHART: MALES | | | |
|---|---|---|---|
| **Guards** | | **Centers and Forwards** | |
| No. of Taps | Score | No. of Taps | Score |
| > 10 | 10 | > 9 | 10 |
| 9 | 8 | 8 | 8 |
| 8 | 6 | 7 | 6 |
| 7 | 4 | 6 | 4 |
| < 6 | 0 | < 5 | 0 |

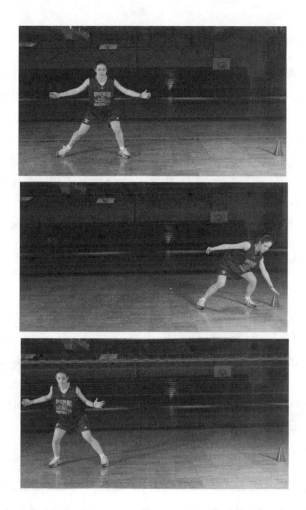

## AGILITY SCORING CHART: FEMALES

| Guards | | Centers and Forwards | |
|---|---|---|---|
| No. of Taps | Score | No. of Taps | Score |
| > 9 | 10 | > 8 | 10 |
| 8 | 8 | 7 | 8 |
| 7 | 6 | 6 | 6 |
| 6 | 4 | 5 | 4 |
| < 6 | 0 | < 5 | 0 |

## Aerobic Fitness

**PURPOSE:** Aerobic fitness enhances the body's efficiency in providing oxygen-rich blood to exercising muscles, aids in recovery following exercise, and prepares the body for more intense training.

Two evaluation techniques are described below: Option 1 is the 1.5-mile run. Option 2 is the step test. Select one based on your preference and convenience. I recommend that the initial test chosen be used for all subsequent evaluations.

### OPTION 1: 1.5-MILE RUN

**TOOLS:** Stopwatch

**TECHNIQUE:** For ease of measurement, conduct this test on a 400-meter (1/4-mile) track. It's a good idea to run this distance as a trial a few days before the evaluation so an efficient and productive pace can be established.

Time how long it takes to run a mile and a half. This is six laps on a 400-meter track.

**SCORING.** Use the following chart to score the 1.5-mile run.

| AEROBIC FITNESS SCORING: 1.5-MILE RUN | | | |
|---|---|---|---|
| **Males** **Time in Minutes** | **Points** | **Females** **Time in Minutes** | **Points** |
| < 8:37 | 10 | < 11:50 | 10 |
| 8:38 to 9:40 | 8 | 11:51 to 12:29 | 8 |
| 9:41 to 10:48 | 6 | 12:30 to 14:30 | 6 |
| 10:49 to 12:10 | 4 | 14:31 to 16:54 | 4 |
| 12:11 to 15:30 | 2 | 16:55 to 18:30 | 2 |
| > 15:31 | 0 | > 18:31 | 0 |

## OPTION 2: STEP TEST

**TOOLS:** 8-inch step, stopwatch

**TECHNIQUE:** This test evaluates recovery heart rate, which is an indicator of cardiovascular efficiency.

Although some versions of this test call for a 12- to 18-inch step, this may be difficult for shorter players or cause pain around the kneecap. I recommend an 8-inch step. This can be in the form of a small single-use box or a long version that several athletes can use at one time.

Keeping the back straight, the athlete should step up with one foot then the other, then down with one foot then the other.

Keep a cadence of 24 steps per minute. This can be paced using a metronome. Each time the metronome clicks a step up or down will be made with each foot.

The test will last for 3 minutes.

Sit down immediately after the test

At 1 minute after the test take the pulse in either the neck or the wrist for 15 seconds. Multiply this number by 4 to calculate your recovery heart rate.

**SCORING.** Use the following charts to score the step test.

| AEROBIC FITNESS SCORING: STEP TEST | | | |
|---|---|---|---|
| Male Heart Rate in | Points | Female Heart Rate in | Points |
| 72 bpm | 10 | 82 bpm | 10 |
| 72 to 76 bpm | 8 | 82 to 90 bpm | 8 |
| 78 to 82 bpm | 6 | 92 to 96 bpm | 6 |
| 84 to 88 bpm | 4 | 98 to 102 bpm | 4 |
| 88 bpm and above | 0 | 102 bpm and above | 0 |

\* Beats Per Minute (bpm)

## Muscle Endurance

**PURPOSE:** Muscle endurance tests are an indicator of how well muscles can sustain long periods of work. The abdominal muscles are evaluated because of their role in maintaining posture and preventing lower back conditions.

**TOOLS:** None.

**TECHNIQUE:** The athlete lays on the floor, knees bent, and hands behind the head. A partner holds the athlete's feet.

During the sit-up, the neck should be kept straight. Exhale when lifting the body. *Do not hold your breath!* A complete repetition is when the elbows touch the knees.

The athlete will complete as many *proper* sit-ups in 1 minute as possible.

**SCORING.** Use the following chart to score muscle endurance.

| MUSCLE ENDURANCE SCORING | | | |
|---|---|---|---|
| **Males** No. of Sit-Ups | **Points** | **Females** No. of Sit-Ups | **Points** |
| > 47 | 10 | > 43 | 10 |
| 43 to 47 | 8 | 39 to 43 | 8 |
| 37 to 42 | 6 | 33 to 38 | 6 |
| 33 to 36 | 4 | 29 to 32 | 4 |
| < 33 | 0 | < 29 | 0 |

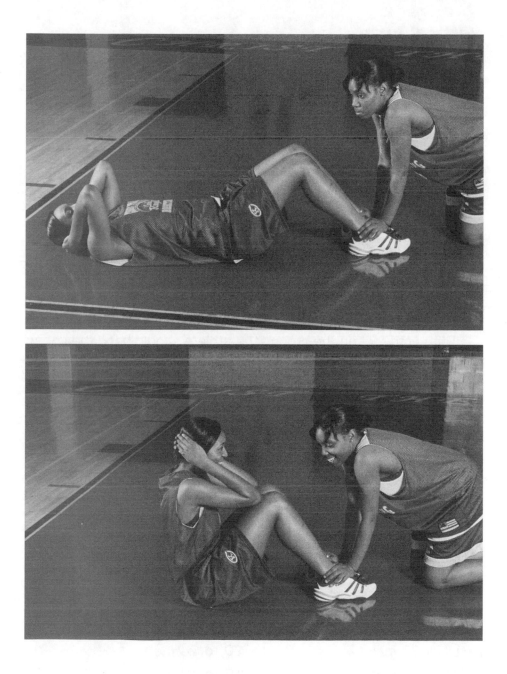

## Vertical Jump

**PURPOSE:** The vertical jump test measures the athlete's ability to jump as if reaching for a rebound, making a block, lay-up, or even a slam-dunk. The greater the height the greater the opportunity to execute these valuable skills in a game.

**TOOLS:** Commercial devices that measure vertical jump height are available for purchase from most sporting goods stores. A less expensive option is to mark the wall from the floor up. For the first seven feet, mark 1-foot intervals. From 7 feet to 12 feet, mark in 1-inch intervals.

**TECHNIQUE:** The athlete stands with his or her dominant side facing the wall. He or she then reaches—from a standing position and without jumping—to the highest point possible.

With both feet on the ground the athlete should bend the knees and swing his or her arms. When ready, have the athlete jump as high as he or she can, reaching for the highest point possible.

When the athlete reaches the highest point an assistant will measure that point. The athlete will repeat this three times and the best trial of the three will be recorded.

**SCORING.** Use the following chart to score the verticle jump test.

| VERTICAL JUMP SCORING | | | | |
|---|---|---|---|---|
| **Males** **Height** | **Points** | **Females** **Height** | | **Points** |
| > 30 inches | 10 | > 25 inches | | 10 |
| 25 to 29 inches | 8 | 20 to 24 inches | | 8 |
| 20 to 24 inches | 6 | 15 to 19 inches | | 6 |
| < 15 inches | 0 | < 10 inches | | 0 |

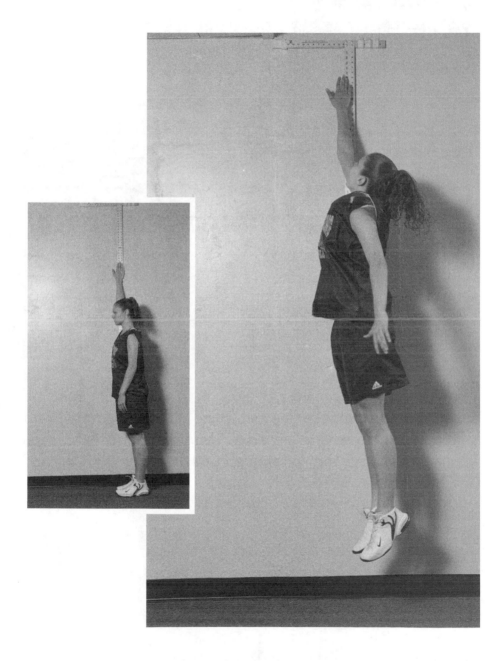

## 3/4-Court Sprint

**PURPOSE:** This test evaluates short burst speed.

**TOOLS:** Stopwatch

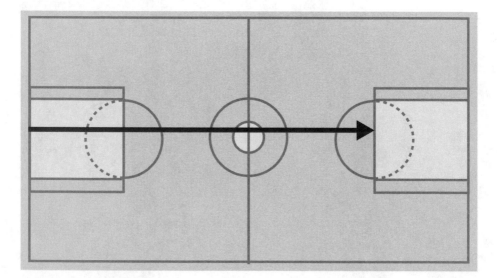

**TECHNIQUE:** The athlete performs an all-out sprint from the baseline to the opposite free throw line while being timed with a stopwatch. The athlete should be instructed to "run through" the free throw line and not stop abruptly.

**SCORING.** Use the following charts to score the 3/4-court sprint test.

## 3/4-COURT SPRINT SCORING: MALES

| Guards | Points | Centers and Forwards | Points |
|---|---|---|---|
| < 3.2 sec. | 10 | < 3.5 sec. | 10 |
| 3.3 to 3.5 sec. | 8 | 3.6 to 3.8 sec. | 8 |
| 3.6 to 3.8 sec. | 6 | 3.9 to 4.1 sec. | 6 |
| 3.9 to 4.0 sec. | 4 | 4.2 to 4.3 sec. | 4 |
| > 4 sec. | 0 | > 4.3 sec. | 0 |

## 3/4-COURT SPRINT SCORING: FEMALES

| Guards | Points | Centers and Forwards | Points |
|---|---|---|---|
| < 3.5 sec. | 10 | < 4 sec. | 10 |
| 3.6 to 3.8 sec. | 8 | 4.1 to 4.4 sec. | 8 |
| 3.9 to 4.1 sec. | 6 | 4.5 to 4.8 sec. | 6 |
| 4.2 to 4.4 sec. | 4 | 4.9 to 5.1 sec. | 4 |
| > 4.5 sec. | 0 | > 5.3 sec. | 0 |

## Full-Court Shuttle

**PURPOSE:** Full-court shuttles, traditionally called "suicides," measure the athlete's anaerobic conditioning, which is the ability to sustain intense efforts on the basketball court.

**TOOLS:** Stopwatch.

**TECHNIQUE:** The full-court shuttle is an all-out sprint. Starting at the baseline, the athlete sprints, without stopping:

**1.** to the near free-throw line;
**2.** back to the starting baseline;
**3.** to the mid court line;
**4.** back to the starting baseline;
**5.** to the far free-throw line;
**6.** back to the starting baseline;
**7.** to the far baseline; and then
**8.** back—and through—the starting baseline

Each time the athlete reaches a baseline, free-throw line, or mid-court line, he or she must tap it.

**SCORING.** Use the following charts to score the full-court shuttle test.

### FULL-COURT SPRINT SCORING: MALES

| Guards | Points | Centers and Forwards | Points |
|---|---|---|---|
| < 26.5 sec. | 10 | < 27.5 sec. | 10 |
| 2.6 to 27.9 sec. | 8 | 27.5 to 28.9 sec. | 8 |
| 28 to 29.9 sec. | 6 | 29 to 30.9 sec. | 6 |
| 30 to 31.9 sec. | 4 | 31 to 32.9 sec. | 4 |
| 32 to 33.9 sec. | 2 | 33 to 34.9 sec. | 2 |
| > 4.4 sec. | 0 | > 52 sec. | 0 |

### FULL-COURT SPRINT SCORING: FEMALES

| Guards | Points | Centers and Forwards | Points |
|---|---|---|---|
| < 28 sec. | 10 | < 30 sec. | 10 |
| 28.5 to 29.9 sec. | 8 | 30.5 to 31.9 sec. | 8 |
| 30 to 31.5 sec. | 6 | 32 to 33.9 sec. | 6 |
| 31.6 to 33.9 sec. | 4 | 34 to 35.9 sec. | 4 |
| 34 to 35.9 sec. | 2 | 36 to 37.9 sec. | 2 |
| > 36 sec. | 0 | >38 sec. | 0 |

## Muscular Strength

**PURPOSE:** Muscular strength is evaluated to determine the athlete's strength capabilities and how these capabilities can be developed to prevent injuries and enhance performance. Two exercises are included: the bench press and the squat.

**OPTION 1: BENCH PRESS**

**TOOLS:** Bench press bench, 2 spotters

**TECHNIQUE:** The athlete lays on the bench with knees bent and feet on the floor. There should be a spotter on each side of the bar. The athlete grabs the bar just wider than shoulder width. When ready, the athlete tells the spotters he or she is ready for

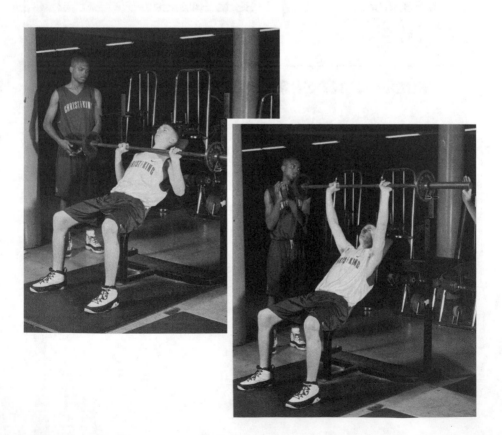

the lift. The athlete lifts the bar from the bench while the spotters have their hands ready beneath the ends of the bar.

The athlete will lower the bar to the chest and raise the arms to an extended position for one good repetition. Be sure to exhale when pushing the bar up. The spotters will assist the athlete in bringing the bar back to the bench supports. The athlete will lift a weight that he or she can lift for only one repetition. This is referred to as the one repetition maximum. In order to safely apply this method the athlete should have been lifting weights for a few weeks.

Prior to the maximum lift attempt execute 10 repetitions as a warm up with a light weight.

It may take a few attempts until the maximum weight is found. Rest 2 to 3 minutes between attempts to let the muscles recover. Record the maximum lift and calculate the percent of the lift compared to the athlete's body weight.

**SCORING:** Use the following chart to score the bench press.

| MUSCLE STRENGTH SCORING OPTION 1: BENCH PRESS | | | |
|---|---|---|---|
| **Males**<br>**% of Body Weight** | **Points** | **Females**<br>**% of Body Weight** | **Points** |
| > 100% | 10 | > 90% | 10 |
| 80 to 90% | 8 | 70 to 80% | 8 |
| 60 to 70% | 6 | 50 to 60% | 6 |
| 40 to 50% | 4 | 30 to 40% | 4 |
| < 40% | 0 | < 30% | 0 |

## OPTION 2: SQUATS

**TOOLS:** Weight belt, squat rack, squat bar

**TECHNIQUE:** For protection, the athlete should wear a weight belt while performing a squat. The athlete stands with the bar resting on his or her shoulders and gripping the bar just wider than the shoulders. Feet will be just wider than shoulder width apart. The back should be kept straight and head and eyes looking slightly up. There should be a spotter on each side of the bar.

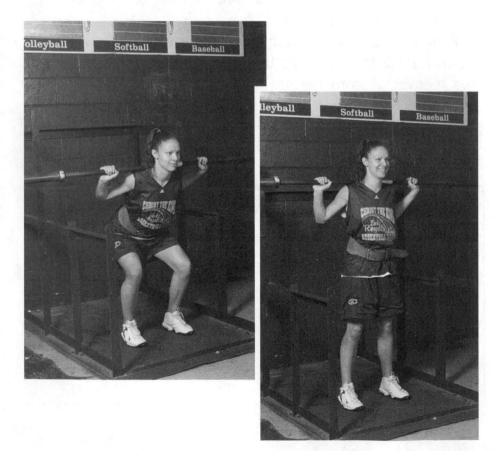

The athlete disengages the bar from the rack.

The athlete will descend into a squat to the point where the thighs are parallel to the ground. Spotters should pay attention to the athlete in case he or she needs assistance. Be sure to exhale when rising with the bar. Upon completing the lift the athlete will step toward the rack and, with the aid of the spotters, place the bar back onto the rack.

The athlete will squat and rise with a weight they can lift only one time. This is referred to as a one repetition maximum. In order to safely apply this method, it's recommended that the athlete lift weights for a few weeks prior to the test session.

Prior to the maximum lift attempt warm up for ten repetitions with a light weight. It may take a few attempts to find the one repetition maximum weight. Rest 2 to 3 minutes between trials. Record the maximum one-repetition lift and calculate its percentage of the athlete's body weight.

| MUSCLE STRENGTH SCORING OPTION 2: SQUATS | | | |
|---|---|---|---|
| **Males**<br>**% of Body Weight** | **Points** | **Females**<br>**% of Body Weight** | **Points** |
| > 200% | 10 | > 170% | 10 |
| 170 to 190% | 8 | 140 to 160% | 8 |
| 140 to 160% | 6 | 110 to 130% | 6 |
| 110 to 130% | 4 | 80 to 100% | 4 |
| < 110% | 0 | < 80% | 0 |

# Chapter 3

# Principles of Basketball Nutrition

Your efforts in the weight room and on the basketball court require fuel. Bodies are like high-performance cars: They may run if you put regular unleaded fuel in the tank. But they run even better with high octane.

Unfortunately, high school athletes often ignore the value of good nutrition. And they're not the only ones: Nearly 40 percent of American teenagers are overweight. This is due in large part to a diet high in fat and the consumption of empty calories found in soft drinks and candies. Not surprisingly, there are even high school basketball players—boys and girls—who are playing overweight.

This problem is compounded by the irregularity in which teens consume nutritious foods. Many high school students have a doughnut or sweetened cereal for breakfast—if they have breakfast at all. Lunch may be fast food, soda, and a bag of chips. Kids with working parents may frequently rely on fast foods for dinner. In the long-term, this cycle contributes to poor eating habits that can dramatically affect performance on the basketball court, as well as increase the risk of diabetes and heart disease.

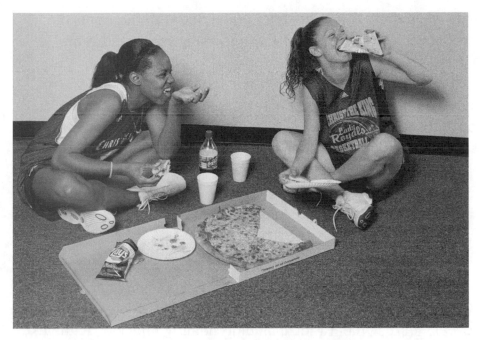

We can't place the burden of poor nutrition exclusively on the shoulders of the athletes. Many health professionals and coaches don't fully understand and appreciate the direct influence diet has on performance. If they do, they may not know how to develop a realistic and comprehensive nutrition program.

Many diet books provide healthy meal options and recipes to follow. Yet many of these programs are not cost effective or logistically feasible for the high school athlete, who typically has very little time (or inclination) to prepare meals. Unless healthy options are readily available, accessible and palatable they are likely to fall by the wayside.

The school environment also plays a role. School food services try to provide nutritious meals, but the odds are often stacked against them. If there is a competing snack bar on school premises or an "open campus" policy that allows students to leave the school property for lunch, there's little doubt about where students end up: the local fast food establishment. While there, students are bombarded with the opportunity to "super size" menu items, consuming more and more of what is least best for them.

Fortunately, there are nutritious choices the high school basketball player can explore to manage weight, maintain or even enhance performance, and prevent short and long-term diet related medical disorders.

# Calorie Consumption

Here is a quick overview of the target calorie consumption for the typical high school athlete.

The average male athlete of high school age consumes 2800 to 3000 calories per day, averaging between 800 and 900 calories per meal (not including healthy snacks). Female athletes should consume approximately 2100 to 2500 calories per day, averaging 600 to 700 calories per meal.

Of these calories, 60 percent should be complex carbohydrates, which provide an efficient fuel source. Approximately 15 to 20 percent of total calories should be from protein, which serves as the "building block" of muscles and connective tissues. For the most part, the "normal" American diet meets this protein requirement, rendering protein supplements unnecessary. Fats, predominately unsaturated, should comprise 25 percent of the diet. Although fat has become the enemy of many diet programs, it too is an excellent source of fuel for the body. The problem arises when too many calories, of any source, are consumed and not stored or metabolized for energy. This will contribute to an increase in body fat.

## FOOD GROUP DAILY SERVINGS

**FATS, OILS, AND SWEETS.** Use sparingly.

**MILK, YOGURT, AND CHEESE.** At least 3 servings a day. 1 serving equals 1 cup of milk or yogurt; 1 1/2 ounces natural cheese; 2 ounces processed cheese.

**MEAT, POULTRY, FISH, BEANS, EGGS, AND NUTS.** Two to 3 servings a day. 1 serving equals 2 to 3 ounces cooked lean meat, poultry, or fish; 1/2 cup cooked dry beans; 1 egg.

**VEGETABLES.** Three to 5 servings a day.

**FRUITS.** Two to 4 servings a day.

**BREADS, CEREAL, RICE, AND PASTA.** Six to 11 servings.

## Fats

To maintain a healthy diet, try to eat unsaturated fats. Most forms of food contain some degree of fat. Try to limit the amount of fat in your diet by eliminating foods that have more than 3 grams of fat per one hundred calories, for example a double cheeseburger with special sauce. In most fast food restaurants, this means staying below 20 grams of fat.

Also try to avoid what I call "nutritional contradictions." For instance, eating a salad is great, but not if you cover it with lots of ranch or blue cheese dressing. Substitute these fatty dressings with oil and vinegar. Other examples include potatoes with sour cream, or a double cheeseburger with a diet soda. These combinations are only fooling you.

## Vitamins and Minerals

For the most part, healthy high school athletes consume the required levels of vitamins and minerals and may only require a daily multivitamin.

One category the growing athlete does need to consider is calcium. High school students should consume approximately 1200 mg/day. This correlates to four servings from the dairy food group. It's often true that as students consume more soft drinks, calcium absorption goes down. In this case, calcium supplementation may be necessary to ensure proper bone development. Seek medical advice prior to any supplementation.

## Water

As water comprises 60 percent of body weight and 70 percent of muscle, its importance can't be underestimated. Drinking copious amounts of milk and soda will not supply or replenish the necessary hydration levels to maintain athletic function.

Try to avoid caffeinated drinks because of the diuretic effect, which can contribute to dehydration. Your goal should be to drink no less than 3 liters of water per day.

Depending on the athlete, environment, intensity of exercise, and season of the year, you may need to consume more water. Sports drinks are also a good source of carbohydrates and will help to replenish electrolytes lost from excessive sweating. Although sports drinks are useful, and more tasteful than water, use them only as an adjunct source of hydration and not a replacement for water.

# Meal Plans

For many athletes and their families, eating healthy may require changes in behavior, planning, and discipline.

When people say, "Breakfast is the most important meal of the day," they're right. Breakfast should include recommended foods such as pancakes, bagels, oatmeal, unsweetened cereal and/or fruit. Breakfast drinks can also serve as a valuable morning tool.

Skipping breakfast or eating a meal high in simple sugars can result in low blood sugar levels as the morning wears on. This can result in headache, dizziness, and difficulty concentrating through morning classes.

Try a mid-morning healthy snack such as juice and pretzels, popcorn, fruit or cut up vegetables. This will keep you going through the morning, provide added nutrients to the body, help in the digestive process, and decrease the desire to gorge on junk food at lunchtime.

Lunch can include a turkey sandwich, veggie hero, peanut butter and jelly sandwich, juice-water-sport drink, fruit, pretzels or popcorn. This chapter also provides a list of "safe" fast foods for the *occasional* meal. A mid-afternoon snack high in complex carbohydrates such as pretzels or an energy bar with a sport drink and water will provide the fuel necessary to get through practice. Avoid salads and vegetables at this time since this can contribute to bloating and gas during practice. After practice have a complex carbohydrate snack and a sport drink to quickly replenish your energy stores for the next day.

Dinner should be a relaxing and fulfilling experience, in moderation. This

## The following foods are good sources of complex carbohydrates

Bagels
Cheese pizza
Crackers
Fruit yogurt
Fruits
Oatmeal
Pancakes
Pasta
Popcorn
Potatoes
Pretzels
Rice
Unsweetened cereals
Vegetables
Whole wheat bread

## The following foods are good sources of protein

Beans
Cheese
Chicken (skinless)
Eggs
Fish
Lean beef
Lean ham
Peanuts
Skim/low fat milk
Turkey (skinless)

meal further contributes to the energy and vitamin/mineral banks of the body. Broiled-skinless chicken with rice/potato and vegetables is a good start. Pasta with a meat sauce and bread and salad is another way to go.

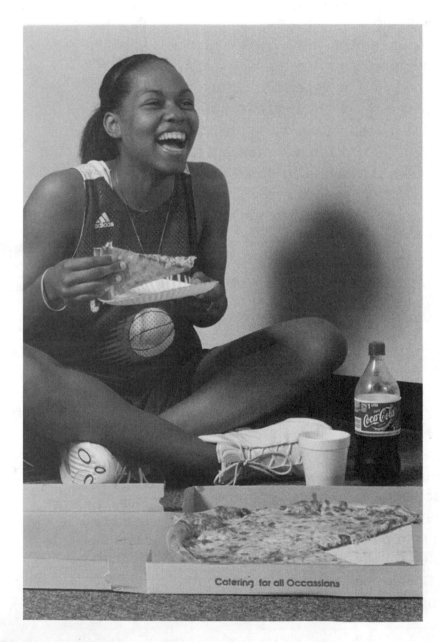

## Smart Fast Food Choices

When pressed for time, the following is a list of popular fast food establishments and foods that will not dramatically hinder athletic performance. It can't be said enough that fast foods should be a last resort and not eaten more than 2 to 3 times per week in total. Avoid "super sizing," "special sauces," mayonnaise, and soft drinks. Limit the amount of fries you eat as well. Some of these items/menus may change following publication of this book. Try to select similar alternatives.

**BURGER KING®**
BK Broiler
Cheese Burger
Chicken Tenders
Hamburger
Small portion of fries

**MCDONALD'S®**
McGrilled Chicken Classic
Hamburger
Cheeseburger
Garden Salad
Chicken McNuggets
Small portion of fries

**PIZZA HUT®**
Ham and Cheese Sandwich
Pan Cheese Pizza
Spaghetti with Meat Sauce
Thin and Crispy Cheese Pizza

**SUBWAY®**
Ham and Swiss
Roast beef
Turkey
Veggie

**TACO BELL®**
Light Chicken Burrito
Light Chicken Taco
Bean Burrito
Beef Burrito
Tostada
Pintos and Cheese

# Quick Energy Sources

After school you may be tired due to lack of sleep or poor nutrition. The normal response is to find a quick boost. But the most important thing to remember about quick energy sources is that there aren't any that are safe or productive. For example:

## Candy

Many chocolate bar companies advertise the quick energy their product will provide when you're dragging. What they don't tell you is that you will get a brief boost in energy from the influx of sugar in the blood stream, which causes the body to release insulin. When the insulin is released you may be dragging more than you were before the candy. This could spell disaster if it's the middle or end of a game or practice.

## Caffeinated Drinks

This can include coffee or the increasing number of super caffeinated soft drinks. Caffeine acts as a diuretic, which increases urinary output. This can contribute to dehydration. Caffeine is also a stimulant that can increase or cause irregular heart rates.

## Weight-Loss Pills and Chinese Herbs

Many of these products include caffeine and the Chinese herb Mahuang-Ephedra. This can be a dangerous combination for athletes who have increased heart rates from exercise. These supplements have been associated with increased and irregular heart rates, strokes, and deaths.

# Managing Your Weight

On those occasions when the athlete may need to gain or lose weight, remember that there are no short cuts. Avoid "weight gain" formulas or supplements or crash diets—losing weight takes time. These methods can negatively affect your performance and are dangerous.

## Gaining Weight

Here are some tips for putting on weight safely.
- Increase caloric intake of healthy foods.
- Eat more healthy snacks during the day.
- Supplement your diet with milkshakes, healthy sandwiches, and pizza.

Weight training is essential at this time to maintain and increase muscle tone, mass, and strength and to ensure that fat levels do not increase.

## Losing Weight

If a responsible health professional determines that weight loss is necessary the process should be gradual, with weight loss not exceeding 2 to 3 pounds per week. Athletes should not reduce their caloric intake below 2000 calories. This would limit the fuel sources necessary to play basketball. The best technique is to reduce back on calories by about 500 per day and increase aerobic activity and weight training. This will ensure that your efforts result in the loss of fat and not muscle or water. Above all else, do not use weight loss pills.

# Injury Nutrition

Nutrition is as important to the injured athlete as it is to the healthy one. When you sprain an ankle or pull a hamstring, the damaged tissues and muscles require specific nutrients to aid in the healing process. Some experts believe that nutrition contributes 25 percent to the healing process.

When sidelined with an injury, you may want to consider decreasing your caloric intake unless you can do substitution exercises such as biking or pool running. If you do not decrease your intake, when you eventually return to play you may be carrying a few unwanted pounds. Maintain healthy snacking, avoiding chips, dips, and sodas. Many of these foods are high in phosphorus, which can deplete calcium levels.

Fried and fatty foods can impair circulation and delay the healing process. While your body heals, circulation cleans out the injury site and provides resources.

If a proper diet is maintained supplementation is usually not required. However, vitamin C is critical to the healing process, contributing to the formation of strong connective tissues. Vitamin C supplements in the range of 500 to 1000 milligrams per day can help as you heal.

# Chapter 4
# Flexibility Training

**S**uccessful basketball players rely on the foundation provided through flexibility training or stretching. Simply defined, flexibility is the ability of a joint to move through a range of motion, for example, in a thigh stretch. Depending on the athlete's flexibility, the heel will be different distances from the buttocks at the maximum point of tension. You can generally determine where you stand in terms of flexibility by performing the pre-season flexibility tests.

Flexibility can be affected by genetics—hypomobile athletes have limited flexibility, while hypermobile athletes appear "double-jointed"—and by inactivity or past injuries.

The benefits of stretching on your performance should not be underestimated. Stretching can increase joint mobility, decrease the risk of injury and post exercise stiffness, as well as contribute to enhanced neuromuscular coordination and efficiency of movement.

To understand the how's and why's of stretching you must understand the function of two receptors in the muscles. The

Golgi Tendon Organ monitors tension generated in the muscle tendon junction. When tension becomes too excessive, the Golgi Tendon virtually shuts the muscle down to protect it from injury. The Muscle Spindle, found within the muscle, monitors excessive rate and length of a stretch put on the muscle. When the Muscle Spindle is stimulated through ballistic stretching a reactive contraction of the muscle occurs, called the Myotatic Stretch Reflex.

Static stretching calls for the limb to be moved to a point where a gentle stretch is experienced on the muscle and there is no pain. Each stretch is held for about 15 seconds and repeated 2 to 3 times. On the other hand, Ballistic stretching is a kind of stretching that involves bouncing motions. The problem with this is that it increases the risk of incurring the Myotatic Stretch Reflex and possible injury to the muscle you arc attempting to stretch.

Static stretching is the safer and preferred form of developing flexibility. Both of the sensors are used successfully in this conditioning technique. When used properly, the Golgi Tendon Organ principle is used in a flexibility technique called Contract-Relax, and the Muscle-Spindle is used in the power development technique called Plyometrics (to be discussed later).

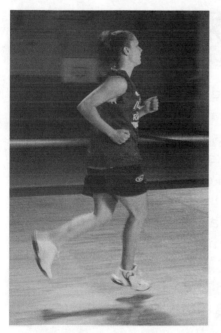

Although elastic in nature, muscles will use their plastic properties to develop improvements in flexibility by developing a memory of elongation as a result of the appropriate program.

It is through static stretching that long-term flexibility benefits can effectively and safely be achieved.

Before stretching warm up for about five minutes with a jog around the gym or by jumping rope to increase body temperature. The warm-up can increase the safety and effectiveness of the flexibility program by increasing muscle temperature and circulation to the muscle. Warming up muscles in this way has also been shown to enhance nerve transmission and muscle metabolism. The warm-up also provides a psychological benefit to aid in the athlete's mental preparation for practice.

Following practice a cool-down jog or jump rope similar to the warm-up will allow for improved circulation of blood that has been concentrated on the exercising legs. Follow the cool-down with the same stretching routine to decrease the risk of postexercise stiffness, especially in the early days of the season when the athlete has yet to establish that plastic memory in the muscle.

## Application of Static Stretching

1. Stretching should be conducted before and after practices and games throughout the year following a warm-up and cool-down.
2. Start with a five-minute jog around the gym or jump rope for both the warm-up and cool-down.
3. Begin the stretching routine in a team formation determined by the coach. Some coaches prefer a circle, semicircle, columns or a more informal set up where the players choose their position, as long as all players can see the designated leaders. Players should be familiar with the techniques of each stretching exercise. Coaches should

walk around and ensure proper technique. Stretching should not be competitive—athletes with different abilities and should be encouraged to maintain proper form to achieve the best results. Compromising form will not produce results and can cause injury.

4. The athlete should gradually ease into the position without bouncing or stretching to the point of pain.

5. Hold the stretch position for a count of 15. This can be repeated 2 to 3 times.

6. Stretching is an exercise that requires normal respiration. Avoid the tendency to hold your breath.

7. Concentrate on the body part being stretched and the proper technique.

# Calves

While in the push-up position, raise the midsection. The foot of the leg being stretched should be kept on the floor with the heel slightly turned out. The knee should be kept straight but not locked. Place the other foot behind the heel of the leg being stretched to avoid sliding. Do not put the non-stretching foot over the Achilles tendon being stretched since this can impede blood flow in the muscle. Keep the foot of the leg being stretched straight or with the heel slightly turned out. Alternate legs after each count of 15 seconds.

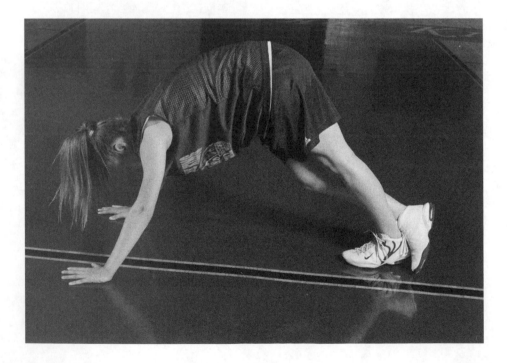

# Hamstrings

Lie flat on your back and lift the leg being stretched. Grab the shin keeping the leg straight but not locked. The leg of the non-stretching knee can be slightly bent. Do not lift the buttocks off the floor or twist the body to reach the leg. If you have difficulty reaching the leg use a towel or band to pull the leg back to the stretch position. This is a preferred method for stretching the hamstrings since it eliminates low back involvement. Alternate legs after each count of 15 seconds.

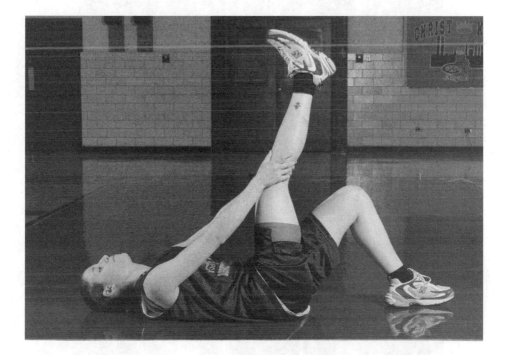

# Quadriceps

While facing each other, two players each grab the ankle of the leg being stretched while balancing with the other hand on the partner's shoulder. Place the heel of the foot close to the buttocks and slowly pull the leg back. Do not grab the foot; this can place stress on the foot and ankle. Alternate after each count of 15 seconds.

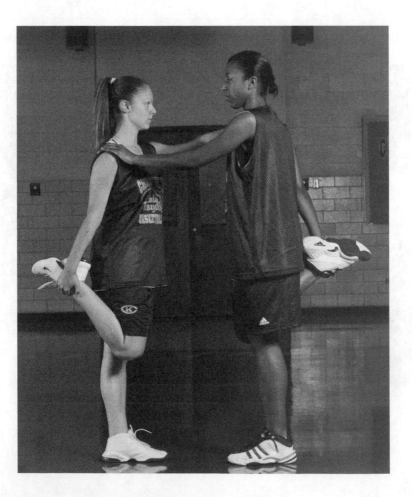

# Adductors

Sit on the floor with the knees bent and the bottom of the feet together. Hold your feet or ankles with your hands and place your elbows on the inside of the thighs. Keeping the back straight, push the legs down while slowly leaning forward.

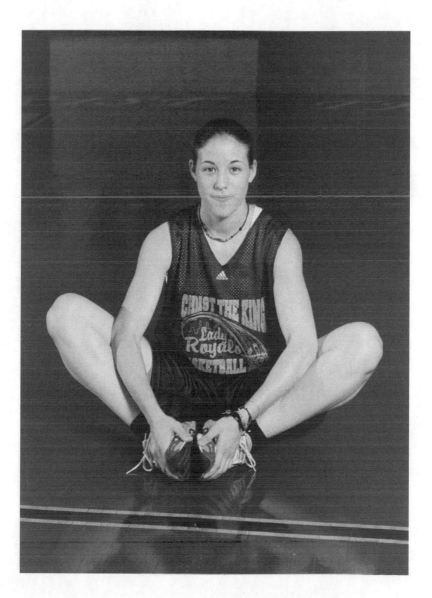

# Iliotibial Band

While standing up, place the leg to be stretched behind the other leg. Tilt the body to the opposite side of the leg being stretched. Alternate legs after each count of 15 seconds.

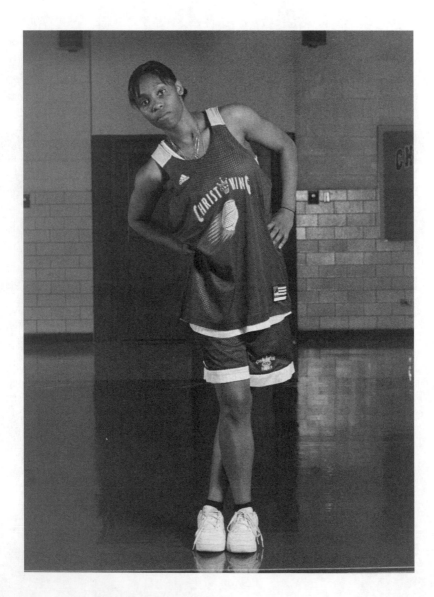

# Hip Flexors

While in a lunge position bend one leg to 90 degrees in front and kneel on the leg being stretched (which should also be flexed to 90 degrees.) Keep the back straight. To perform the stretch on the back leg, move the hip forward while leaning back with your trunk. Alternate legs after each count of 15 seconds.

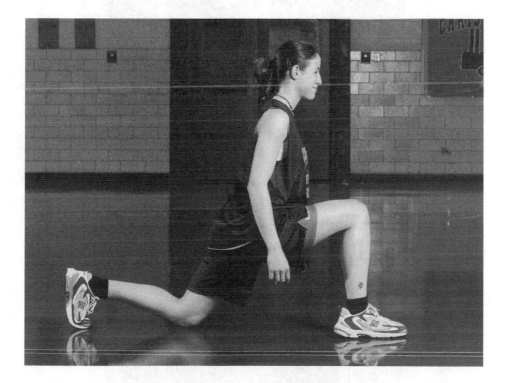

# Lower Back A

While sitting up, place the legs just past shoulder width apart with the knees slightly flexed. Grab the ankles and slowly lean forward while keeping the back straight. After 15 seconds release the stretch, and then repeat.

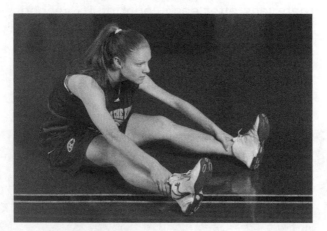

# Lower Back B

Lie on your back and cross your leg over the trunk of your body. Alternate legs after each count of 15 seconds.

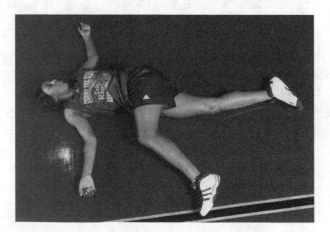

# Neck A

Interlock the fingers behind the head and slowly pull the head forward. Hold the stretch for 15 seconds, release, then repeat.

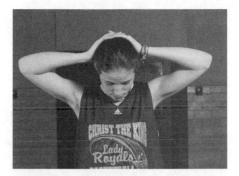

# Neck B

While keeping the shoulders straight grab the right side of the head and pull it slowly to the left. Hold the stretch for 15 seconds, release, then repeat.

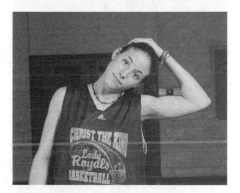

# Neck C

While keeping the shoulders straight grab the left side of the head and pull it to the right. Hold the stretch for 15 seconds, release, then repeat.

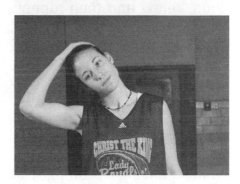

# Shoulders A

While standing up straight pull the arm to be stretched across the chest at shoulder level. Grab the elbow and slowly pull the arm across the chest. Alternate arms after each count of 15 seconds.

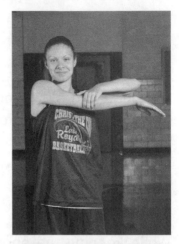

# Shoulders B

While standing up straight, clasp the hands behind the back and slowly lift them up. Hold the stretch for 15 seconds, relax, and then repeat.

# Shoulders C

While standing up straight bend the arm to be stretched over the head with the hand resting between the shoulder blades. Take the other hand and place it on the elbow of the shoulder being stretched and slowly push down. Alternate arms after each.

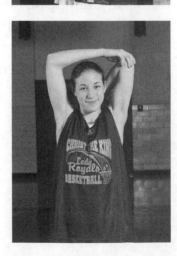

# Wrist Flexors

Start with the hand bent up, held with the other hand and the elbow bent. To stretch the muscle, slowly straighten the elbow. Alternate arms after each count of 15 seconds.

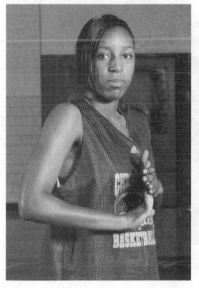
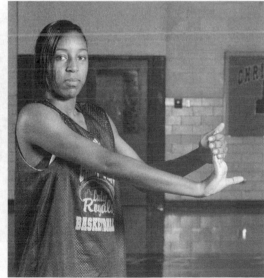

# Wrist Extensors

Start with the wrist bent down, held by the other hand and the elbow bent. To stretch the muscle, slowly straighten the elbow. Alternate arms after each count of 15 seconds.

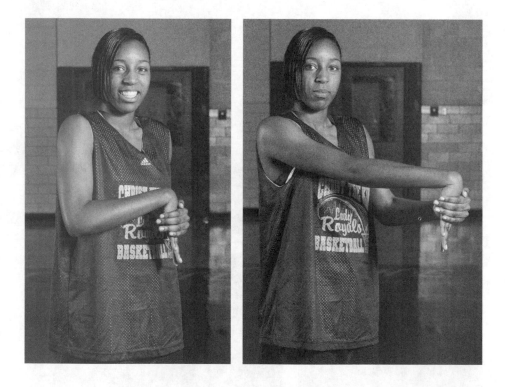

# Contract-Relax Stretching

Contract-Relax stretching is an effective form of stretching which helps develop flexibility, especially for athletes who do not respond to static stretching, who have poor flexibility, or as a valuable adjunct to the static stretching program.

Contract-Relax relies on the properties of the Golgi Tendon Organ. When the muscle is stretched, then contracted isometrically (without movement of the limb), the Golgi Tendon Organ responds by relaxing the tension. The athlete is then able to stretch the muscle further. This form of stretching is also good for those who have poor flexibility and need a "jump start" prior to practice, or for those who become stiff during a game or practice. The following program can be done as an alternative to the previously described Static Stretching program. Warm up prior to Contract-Relax stretching.

## Principles of Contract-Relax

1. It is important in this form of stretching that the partners communicate with each other.
2. The partner will move the limb to a position where a stretch is experienced on the athlete's muscle. The athlete being stretched should tell the partner when a stretch is experienced. At this point the athlete being stretched will isometrically contract the muscle for 10 seconds. For the person being stretched, gradually build up the contraction but avoid rapid movements. This can injure both the person being stretched as well as their partner. After the isometric contraction gradually release the tension on the muscle. The partner briefly relaxes the limb then moves it to the next position of the stretch. Repeat this process three times. After the third repetition relax the limb then bring it to a final position which will be held statically for 15 seconds.

Since the primary muscles involved in basketball are those found in the lower extremities only these groups will be discussed. There are specific techniques for the upper extremities as well.

# Calves

The athlete being stretched will sit on the floor with the back of the knee resting on a basketball. The partner will hold the ankle with one hand while the other hand is on the bottom of the foot slowly pushing it forward. The athlete being stretched will push the foot down during the contraction phase of the stretch. Execute Contract-Relax Technique then alternate legs.

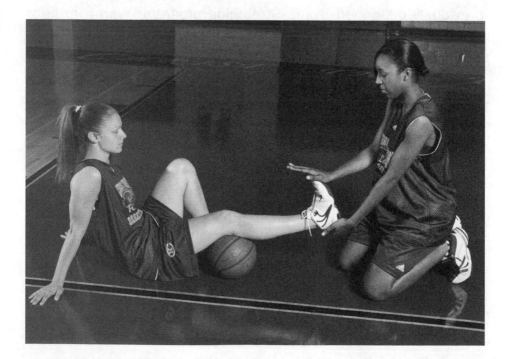

# Hamstrings

The athlete being stretched will lie on his or her back. The leg being stretched will be kept straight but not locked. The partner will lift the leg being stretched into the desired position. The athlete being stretched must concentrate on not lifting the hips off the floor or twisting the hip in any way when performing the contraction. The partner can use his or her shoulder for leverage to hold the stretching leg up while keeping the lower leg from rising. To perform the contraction, the athlete being stretched will push the raised leg forward. Execute the Contract-Relax technique then alternate legs.

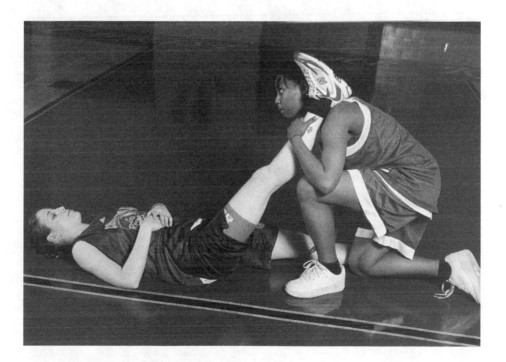

# Quadriceps

With the athlete being stretched lying on his or her stomach the partner should slowly bend the leg bringing the heels towards the buttocks. To keep the athlete being stretched from raising the hips, the partner can hold the leg being stretched with either his or her hand or shoulder and hold the hip of the stretching side with the opposite hand. The athlete being stretched will attempt to push their foot toward the floor. Execute the Contract-Relax technique then alternate legs.

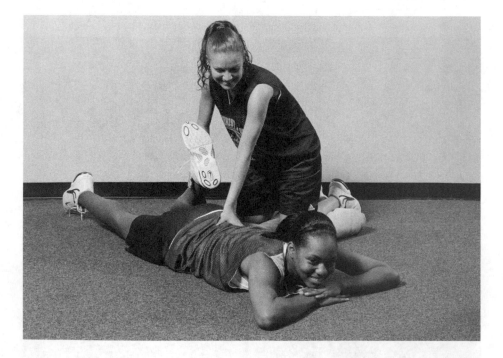

# Adductors

The athlete being stretched will sit up with knees bent and bottom of the feet together bringing the heels close to the body and keeping the back straight. The partner will kneel facing the athlete placing his or her hands on the inside of the knees of the athlete being stretched. The athlete being stretched will contract by pushing the knees up into the partner's hands. Execute Contract-Relax technique with both legs worked on simultaneously.

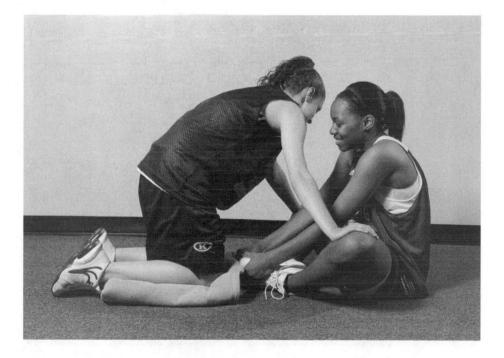

# Iliotibial Band

The athlete being stretched will lie on his or her back. The leg of the hip being stretched will be bent to 90 degrees with the foot placed on the outside of the non-stretching leg, which is kept flat. The partner will kneel on the side of the leg being stretched placing one hand on the shoulder and the other on the outside of the knee of the hip being stretched. The contract phase will occur with the athlete being stretched pushing the outside of the knee into the hand of the partner. The athlete being stretched should keep the bent leg foot on the floor, not lift the hips or twist the back. Execute Contract-Relax technique then alternate legs.

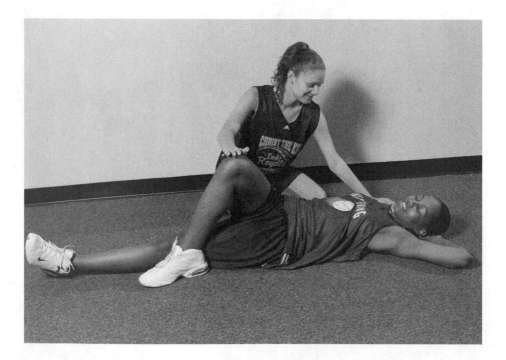

# Hip Flexors

With the athlete being stretched lying on his or her stomach keep the knee bent to about 90 degrees. The partner will kneel on the outside of the leg being stretched putting one hand on the hip and the other holding up the thigh. The contraction phase will occur with the athlete being stretched pushing the thigh toward the ground. Execute the Contract-Relax technique then alternate legs.

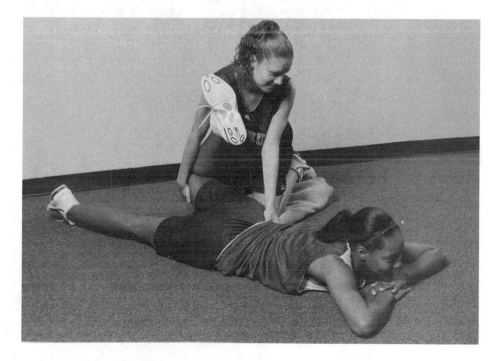

# Lower Back

The athlete being stretched will be sitting up with the legs partially flexed and the feet just past shoulder width apart. The partner will be behind, placing his hands on the shoulder blades. The contract phase occurs with the athlete being stretched pushing back into the partner's hands. The athlete being stretched should not lift the body off of the floor. Execute Contract-Relax Technique.

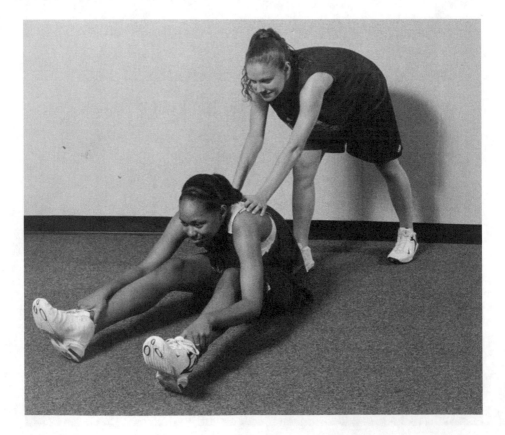

# Chapter 5

# Coordination and Agility Training

It's generally accepted that endurance, flexibility, and strength are the cornerstones of a sound training program. Coordination and agility training is a vital component for any training program, especially for basketball, a multi-directional sport that requires quick stop and go action and reaction as well as changes in body direction—with the feet on and off the ground. The training covered in this chapter provides the glue for efficient neuromuscular performance, as well as helping to prevent injuries and rehabilitate existing injuries. The basic component of coordination is proprioception, the body's radar and initial response system. Receptors found in the muscles, ligaments, and joints monitor and control body position, motion, and tissue stress. They provide muscular reflexes and postural responses to body/limb position and motion. A classic example is the body's ability to catch itself before a fall, for example as you're about to twist your ankle when coming down from a shot or rebound.

While you're playing, these receptors work in conjunction with sight and the balance mechanism found in the inner ear. When called into action, sensory information is transmitted to the central nervous system where it's processed for the appropriate response.

The efficiency of this system, like the others in the body, is determined by the individual's medical history, level of conditioning and physical training.

Recurring injuries can be the result of insufficient training of the proprioceptors. If there's swelling, muscle weakness or ligament laxity following an injury, it's especially important for joint reactions to be regained. Studies have found that knee joint swelling can impede reflex quadriceps contractions, thereby decreasing the potential for regaining strength. It has also been found that decreased proprioceptive capabilities can contribute to degenerative changes in joints.

On a higher level of neuromuscular function, and critical for basketball, is agility. This is the body's ability to quickly change speed and direction.

Athletes who appear clumsy, particularly high school or middle school athletes, can greatly benefit from this type of training. Without coordination training, the teenager's inability to adjust to rapid growth spurts can frustrate coach and athlete alike. Even though height is a definite advantage for a basketball player, it isn't everything. A well-coordinated shorter player can run circles around a taller gawky player. What counts is the efficiency with which the athlete's resources are utilized, and this is especially relevant for a multi-directional sport such as basketball.

Despite the apparent simplicity of these exercises, their value is immeasurable. They serve as the precursor to sport-specific agility drills applied at practice. Some of these exercises will be done with your eyes open and closed, since body adjustment and reaction time in sports is not always dependent on visual cues. Information collected by the brain during these exercises is stored for later use. It is also recommended that these exercises be done before a workout as fatigue can affect the effectiveness of the results.

The beauty of coordination and agility exercises is that they don't rely upon expensive equipment to effectively develop this body system. Start with the first exercise and progress to the next drill only when proficiency has been achieved. These aren't as easy as they appear. Jumping too far forward, as with any training program, can impede development and result in injury. This routine can be incorporated into your regular training program.

The ultimate goal of these exercises is to further challenge the athlete in a sport specific manner. Coaches have their own creative methods and tools, and these exercises serve as a foundation for the coach's unique program. All these drills can be conducted daily. Some coaches opt to incorporate them at the beginning or end of practice. You can also rotate exercises to avoid staleness and boredom. In any event some form of coordination and agility training needs to be done daily.

# Single-Leg Stand I

Stand on one leg with both hands on the hips and eyes open. Attempt to hold this position for a count of 10 and repeat five to 10 times. Repeat the process on the other leg. Work up to holding the position for 15 seconds. Now, do the same exercise with your eyes closed.

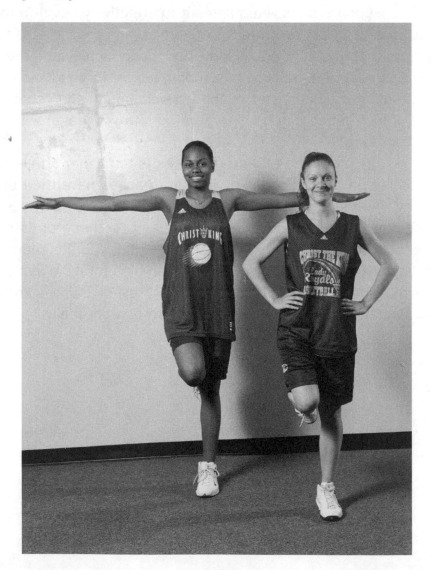

# Single-Leg Stand II

Stand on one leg with arms at shoulder level and your eyes open (see picture on page 84). Attempt to hold this position for a count of 10 and repeat five to 10 times. Repeat this process on the other leg. Work up to holding the position for 15 seconds. Now, do the same exercise with your eyes closed.

The foot must remain stable during the two previous exercises, with no shuffling or twisting of the leg and body. Try not to lose your balance to the point of falling down, but don't get discouraged if at first you can't hold the 10-second position. Hold for as long as you can, repeat the exercise and keep trying. These simple, yet important exercises can be incorporated into the warm-up or post practice stretch session and should be done every day.

For more of a challenge the athlete can progress to a wobble board where they attempt to keep the sides from hitting the ground, or a mini-trampoline. Again attempt to hold for a count of 10 and repeat five to 10 times before switching to the other leg. Eventually work up to holding the position for 15 seconds. Make sure to do the exercise with your eyes open and closed.

# Cross-Crawl Strides

Cross-Crawl strides can be used as a functional warm-up drill while at the same time helping to develop coordination. Here's how it works. The athlete strides down the court emphasizing lifting one arm and the opposite leg. For example, when the left arm goes up so should the right leg—then alternate while progressing down the court and back. It's interesting to observe athletes when they do this drill, as the same arm and leg have a tendency to go up together. The Cross-Crawl pattern develops a connection between one side of the brain and the other side of the body and helps build coordination.

The development of functional coordination and agility involves modified activities that simulate many of the body motions common to basketball.

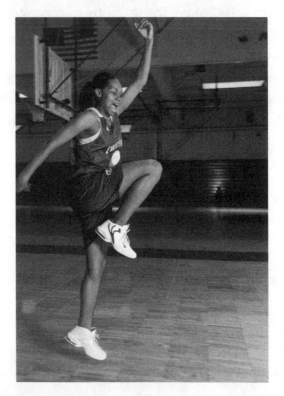

# Box Hops

Box hops involve taping four connected boxes on the floor, each measuring two feet square. With the feet together, hop clockwise into each box for 15 seconds then counter clockwise for fifteen seconds. This can be repeated two to three times, alternating between direction patterns.

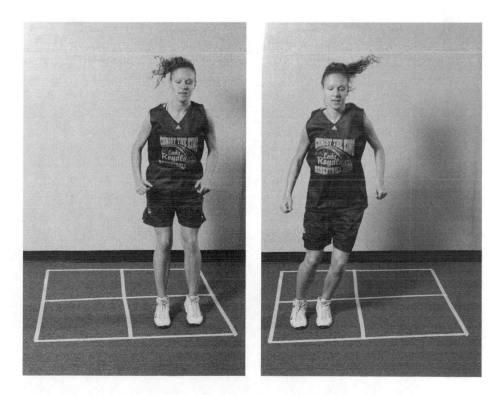

# Dot Board

Dot board requires painting four dots on the floor three feet apart and one in the middle. (Commercially made mats can also be used.) Start with both feet on the middle dot. On "GO" quickly move both feet to the top left dot, then quickly return to the middle dot, quickly move to the top right dot, return to the middle dot, move to the lower left dot, back to the middle and then to the lower right dot. Repeat this process for thirty seconds. This can be repeated two to three times.

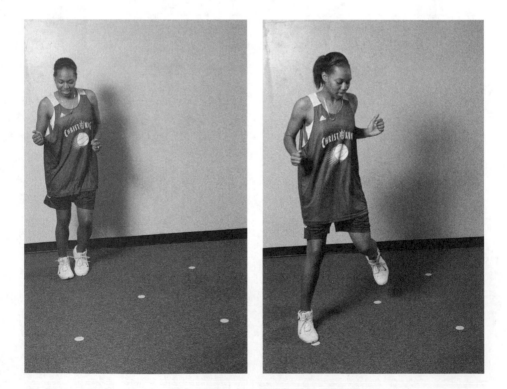

# Agility Ladder

Agility Ladder is a rope ladder with flat rungs. Once again the exercise design is limited only by your imagination. The key is to move the feet quickly through the ladder spaces without hitting the rungs. Some exercises include a side-to-side foot shuffle. While facing forward quickly move both feet into a rung space, then quickly move them both back into the previous space, move both feet forward two spaces, then back one. Repeat this sequence until you have gone through the whole ladder. Another exercise requires alternating one foot in and one foot out progressing up the length of the ladder.

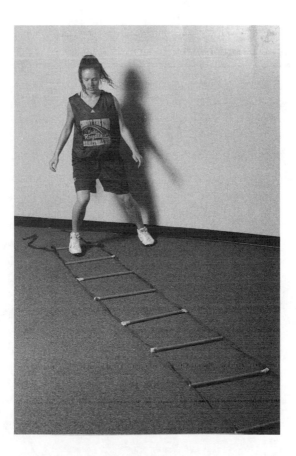

# Run / Shuffle

Within small spaces, the Run/Shuffle can start on the left foul lane on the baseline. Run forward up to the foul line, then sidestep shuffle to the right foul lane, back pedal to the baseline and side step shuffle to the starting point. Repeat as desired or for specified time periods, i.e. 30 to 45 second repeats. In a larger space, start in the left corner of the court on the baseline, run forward to mid court, sidestep shuffle to the right sideline, run backwards to the baseline and end by sidestep shuffling to the left to the beginning point.

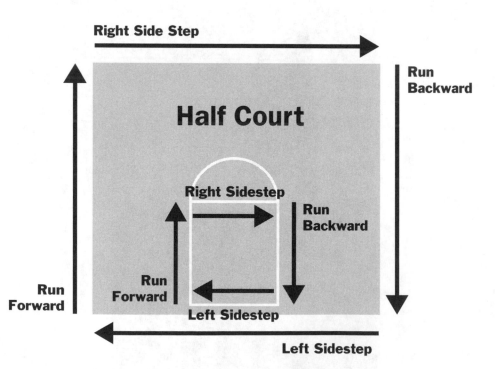

# Carioca

To perform carioca, alternate right foot and left foot cross over starting on the baseline to mid-court. Stay facing the same direction and return to the baseline. This can be progressed to full court up and back.

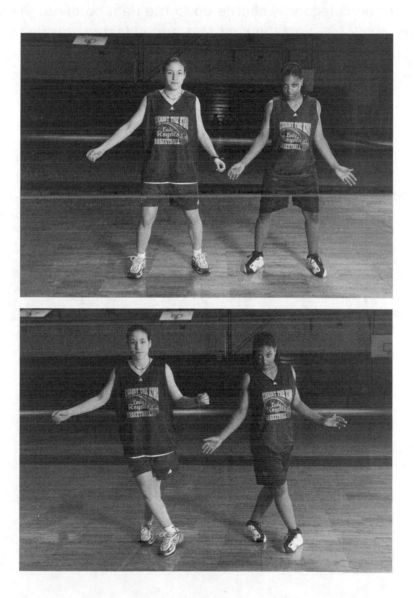

# Shuffle-Pivot X Drill

The Shuffle-Pivot X Drill starts in the left corner of the court on the baseline. While facing out, side step to the mid court line and then back pivot on the right foot. Sidestep diagonally to a cone in the middle of the half court then back pivot off the left foot and diagonally shuffle up to the right corner of the mid court. Back pivot off the right foot and sidestep shuffle to the baseline. Front pivot off the left foot, diagonal sidestep to cone and front pivot on right foot diagonal sidestep back to starting point.

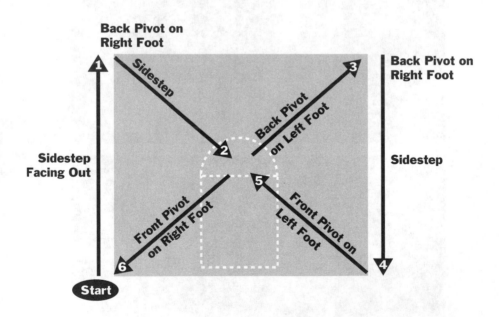

# Zigzag Shuffle

The Zigzag Shuffle starts on the baseline facing diagonally towards the left corner of the court. Sidestep shuffle four steps, back pivot on right foot, sidestep shuffle four steps, and then back pedal on left foot. Repeat process first up to mid-court then full court.

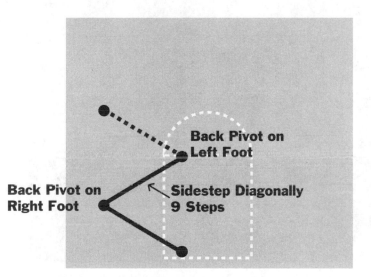

# Upper Body Training

Not to be neglected is the coordination of the arms, elbows, wrists and hands. Although the majority of function and injuries do occur to the lower limbs, the arms undoubtedly play a role in basketball when it comes to catching the ball, shooting the ball and reaching for it. Injuries also occur from falling and being hit by the ball or another player.

# Ball Push-Up

The Ball Push-Up requires balancing on a basketball in the push up position. Hold first then attempt a push-up.

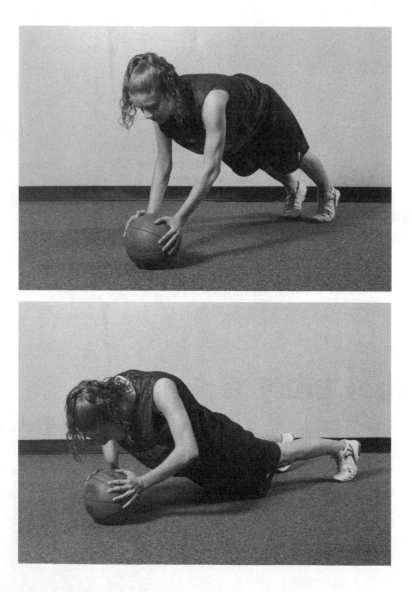

# Chapter 6

# Principles of Strength Training

**S**trength is the body's ability to exert force against resistance. In sports, strength by itself is not nearly as important as the ability to harness strength that can be powerfully exerted in the shortest time possible. A plan to achieve this is one of the athlete's most important training tools and is invaluable to athletic success. In addition to enhancing performance, strength training builds muscle and the connective tissues around joints, decreasing the risk of injury.

Muscles are a network of bundled fibers forming a functioning unit. They range in size from a major muscle group like the quadriceps in the thigh that extend the legs, to the muscles that bend the fingers. The motor nerves from the spinal cord innervate our muscles to form a motor unit, which consists of the nerve and the attached fibers. The muscle is moved in response to a signal received from the brain or spinal cord. To carry out the signal, the necessary amount of motor units is recruited to perform the task.

Muscles also respond to stress. In the case of weight training, the stress is the applied weight. In order to increase strength, the weight must be of a sufficient nature to recruit many motor units. This is the principle behind overload, or lifting more than is customary in daily activities.

As a result of strength training, the muscles will increase in size, a reaction called hypertrophy. There will also be an increased recruitment and coordination of motor units. In this way performance is enhanced, contributing to a greater ability to jump, shoot from further away, set picks, and take charges. Additional benefits of strength training include increased circulation to the muscle and energy stores for future work.

The process of building muscle may take as long as 6 to 8 weeks to firmly take hold. You may see quick gains in strength during the early stages of your program, but this is usually only a neuromuscular response to "wakening the muscles."

Many female athletes are concerned with becoming "muscle bound," but this is virtually impossible due to the smaller amount of the growth hormone testosterone that women possess in comparison to men. Women may find, however, that their clothes fit differently because of their newly developed muscle tone. Improved muscle tone also carries with it the benefit of improved confidence and increased strength.

# Classifications of Weight Training

The demands and skills of specific sports require different applications of weight training. For example, the needs of a basketball forward will be dramatically different from those of a marathon runner. The basketball player needs to develop strength and explosive power to perform short efforts such as jumping for a rebound, while the marathoner requires muscle endurance to cover distances over a prolonged period of time.

Here are some brief descriptions of the basic principles of weight training, along with some tips for getting started.

## Muscle Endurance

Not to be confused with cardiorespiratory endurance, which involves the heart, lungs, and the utilization of oxygen, muscle endurance is the ability of the muscles to contract repeatedly over a long period of time. Muscle endurance forms the foundation to safely transition to higher intensity lifting, and include a muscle endurance program of 1 to 3 sets of 15 repetitions.

## Strength

Strength is the body's ability to exert force against resistance. This can be a weight, another player, or an object such as a ball. Strength is an important ability that serves as the basis of power programs more specifically translated to the basketball court. A strength program would involve 3 sets of 6 to 8 repetitions.

## Power

Power is the ability to take developed strength and exert it explosively in a short matter of time, for example vertical and horizontal jumping ability. Upper body power development will allow you to make and receive sharp passes. The power type of weight lifting will be complemented by power drills to be described in the Power Training Chapter. A power-lifting program would involve 3 sets of 3 to 5 repetitions of a heavier weight.

# Phases of a Lift

**CONCENTRIC PHASE:** During the actual work phase of a lift, the muscle fibers shorten when they contract. This shortening of muscle fibers under tension is called the concentric phase or contraction.

**ECCENTRIC PHASE:** As the limb is returned to the starting position, the motion must be controlled and conducted slowly. During this controlled return, muscle fibers lengthen under tension. This is referred to as the eccentric phase or lengthening. Research has found that more strength can be developed through this phase, making it important to slowly lower the weight. Eccentric contractions are one of the main culprits that contribute to muscle soreness experienced by many athletes in the early stages of a strength program.

# Muscle Soreness

During the early stages of a weight-training program it's normal for an athlete's muscles to become sore and stiff a day or two after working out. For the athlete and parent, this upsetting experience may result in a visit to the doctor. Even if the discomfort is not reduced, the condition is relatively benign in nature, and is not cause for concern. The pain you may experience 24 to 48 hours after a weight-training workout is called Delayed Onset Muscle Soreness (DOMS). For years the cause of DOMS was a matter of debate among exercise specialists. The consensus among contemporary researchers is that DOMS is the result of microscopic tears that occur in the muscles, predominately during the eccentric stage of the lift. These tears subsequently result in swelling and pain. In the case of an acute muscle injury, such as a strain or a tear, the pain is usually instantaneous.

The treatment for DOMS is 15 minutes of ice on the sore area and 30 minutes off, followed by gentle static stretching. You should avoid aggravating activities; however, a light bike ride can loosen you up and ibuprofen can decrease the pain. In a day or two you should be back to normal. Prevention of DOMS includes avoiding heavy weights or numerous sets in the early stages of your program, a good warm up and stretch before the workout, and cool down and stretch afterwards.

# Periodization

Many athletes are under the misconception that if a little training is good, more is better. There's a tendency to want to continuously increase weight in an attempt to get stronger. Eventually you reach the pinnacle of your strength bell curve. If you continue with a linear lifting progression,  you'll find yourself sliding down the other side where the gains you worked for will either stagnate or decrease. This will also increase the risk of physical and emotional burn out.

Therefore, it is important to utilize periodization, a method of breaking up the weight training program into periods of varying levels of intensity, volume, and muscular system training, (i.e. endurance, strength, and power). Periodization can be applied in various ways. For the programs described in this book, the training periods will be designated as off-season, preseason, and in-season.

# De-Training

Weight training is often enthusiastically applied prior to the start of the season. Often, once the season starts, weight room time is dramatically reduced for the sake of skill development. Although skill development is necessary to increase the basketball abilities of the player, if weight training ceases at this time, the gains obtained through your pre season diligence can dissipate by the time it counts most—in conference or postseason play. It has been found that after 8 weeks of not lifting, strength will decrease at least 10 percent and continue from there. This may not seem like much, but it can mean the difference between a win over a team that isn't lifting. To maintain the edge on your competition, an in-season periodization weight training program should be continued.

# Weight Machines vs. Free Weights

The form of resistance training you engage in is often dependent on the resources of your school. For the past ten years, schools throughout the country have recognized the value of weight training and have made a concerted effort to improve their facilities, incorporating cardiovascular equipment, weight machines and free weights. There has also been a growing trend to return to free weight training because of its applicability to sport specific skills. Let's take a look at the two.

## Machines:

- Increase safety because the weights move along a rail. Safety should never be neglected.
- Provide a quick set up. All you need to do is move a bench into position and put the pin securely into the weight rack.
- Allow many athletes to exercise on one multi-station unit in a relatively small space.
- Are often designed to work the muscles according to their force abilities through the range of motion.

## Free Weights:

- Increases neuromuscular coordination.
- Provide the opportunity to work multi-joint power exercises, which are more applicable to athletic performance.
- Increase trunk stabilization.
- Are less expensive than weight machines.

# Safety

Despite the numerous benefits of weight training, a lack of consideration for safety can result in severe injury. The following are safety procedures to follow while in the weight room:

- Avoid running or fooling around.
- Know the proper technique. Don't lock out joints such as your knees and elbows.
- Don't hold your breath.
- Gradually increase weights.
- Have attentive spotters.
- Use weight belts, especially for squats, dead lifts, and shoulder press exercises.
- Use securely fastened collars on all free weight bars.
- Don't leave weights lying on the floor.
- Don't use broken or malfunctioning equipment.
- Be sure that pins are securely placed in weight racks.
- If pain or an injury occurs, stop lifting.
- Wear appropriate clothing (i.e. shorts, sweats, T-shirts, and athletic shoes).
- Don't wear any jewelry.
- Long hair should be tied up.

# PRINCIPLES OF WEIGHT TRAINING

- Warm up, cool down, and stretch before and after each session.
- Follow all safety guidelines.
- Weight training can be conducted 2 to 3 days per week. The programs described in this book involve lifting 2 days per week with 48 hours of recovery. This will allow you to develop strength while having ample time to hone basketball skills. This is also intended to be a more convenient schedule enhancing long-term compliance. Some books describe programs that are time consuming and unrealistic for the high school player and coach. Remember, weight training is an adjunct to success.
- The duration, or number of sets and repetitions, is based upon the program established in the periodization schedule.
- **MUSCULAR ENDURANCE:** 1 to 3 sets of 15 repetitions. Average a 30-second rest between sets. Some coaches prefer a circuit program where the athlete lifts for 30-45 seconds at a particular station then immediately moves to the next station when the time has expired.
- **STRENGTH:** 3 sets of 6 to 8 repetitions with 1 1/2 to 2 minutes rest between sets.
- **POWER:** 3 sets of 3 to 5 repetitions with 2 minute rest between sets.

- **INTENSITY:** for muscular endurance, use a weight that you can lift 15 times. When this becomes easy, increase the weight by no more than 10 pounds, since most weight machines are set at 10-pound intervals.

For strength and power development, the traditional method for determining the appropriate lifting weight is as a percentage of the one repetition maximum, or 1 RM. Although this is an effective method, great care and attention needs to be considered when applying the 1 RM. The athlete should thoroughly warm up, stretch, and complete a warm-up set of 10 repetitions using a light weight. Achieving the 1 RM may take several attempts, which increases fatigue. Keep in mind that fatigue may cloud the true 1 RM. In the rush to find a maximum weight for the 1 RM, an injury may occur. Consider these variables before using this method.

My preferred method for assessing the appropriate exercise weight is to find a weight that can be lifted for the recommended number of repetitions for that day. For instance, if the prescription is for 3 sets of 6 repetitions, find the weight that can be lifted 6 times. The last repetitions should be difficult but not adversely affect your technique. When six repetitions can be completed, increase the weight. This format takes into consideration your abilities for that given day. Using the other method, if you are prescribed to lift a certain percentage of the 1 RM and have difficulty with it, you may become discouraged and attempt a weight that may increase the risk of injury. ■

# Weight Lifting Exercises: Free Weights

You can combine free weights and weight machines into your program. Many of the exercises described in this section can also be combined within your periodization program. For instance, tricep extensions or heel raises on a weight machine may feel more comfortable than free weights.

## WEIGHT LIFTING HINTS AND TIPS

- Follow proper technique for all lifts. If technique is compromised, lower the weight.
- Always lift the weight through the full range of motion.
- Never exercise the same body parts on consecutive days or lift the day before a game. In the conditioning program described later in this book, the in-season program has identified lifting days. You may need to alter this based on your game schedule, but be sure to give yourself at least 24 to 48 hours rest between sessions.
- Avoid excessive increases in weight.
- Maintain proper posture with all exercises.
- Perform the negative lift slowly. The pace can be twice as long as it takes for the concentric phase.
- For most exercises, hands should be placed on the bar approximately shoulder width apart. Feet should also be about shoulder width apart. This will ensure a secure grip and adequate support base.

# Squats

Stand with the bar on your shoulders. A folded towel behind your neck may increase comfort. Hands and feet should be slightly past shoulder width apart, with your feet slightly turned out.

Lower yourself so that your thighs are parallel to the ground, keeping your heels on the floor. Your back should be straight with your head up.

Proper technique is to keep your shoulders over your knees and your knees over your feet. Do not let your knees go beyond your feet.

Spotters can be on both sides of the bar.

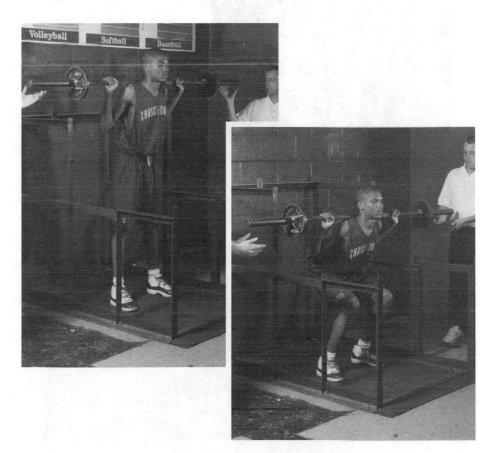

# Lunges

Hold two dumbbells in each hand or a barbell on your shoulders. Take a step forward, bending your front leg to a 90 percent angle. Keeping your back straight, look forward and do not let your knee extend beyond your foot.

Return to the starting position and alternate feet.

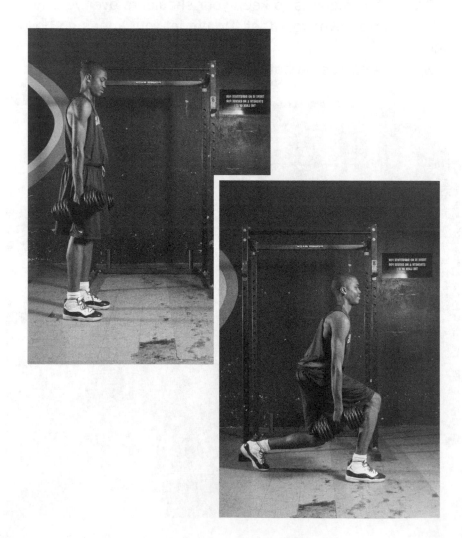

# Heel Raises

Stand with the front of your feet on a board 2 to 3 inches high. Place the bar on your shoulders, gripping it just past shoulder width apart. Keep your back and knees straight, but not locked.

Rise up on your heels.

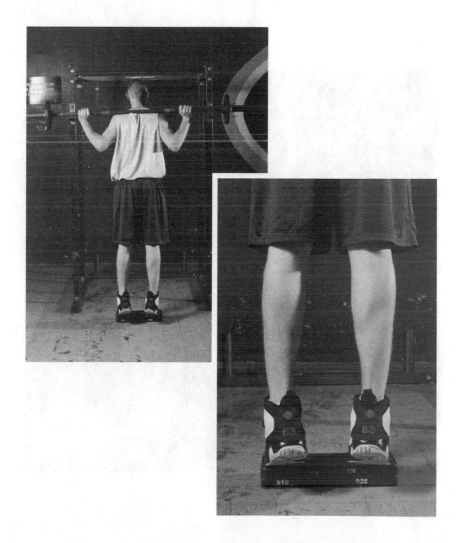

# Bench Press

For basketball training, an incline bench is preferred.

Lie on your back, placing your hands on the barbell just past shoulder width apart and bring the bar to the chest. Lift the bar by extending, not locking your elbows. Bring the bar back to the starting position. Keep your back flat on the bench at all times.

Spotters can be on both sides of the bar or behind you.

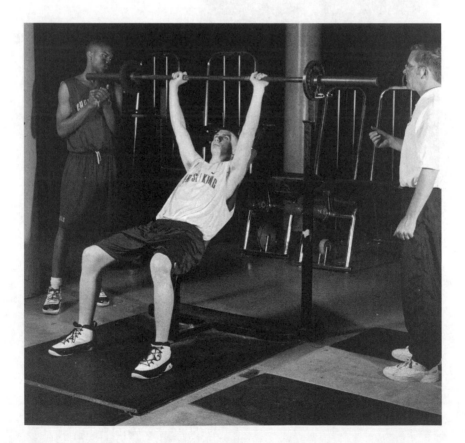

# Rows

Bend at the waist over the bar and grip it just past shoulder width apart. Lift the bar to your chest.

Do not pull the weight up with your lower back.

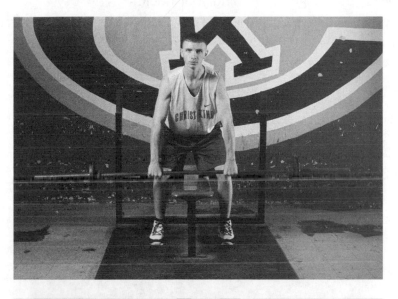

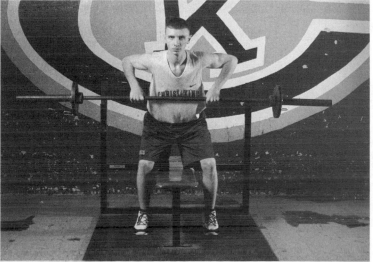

# Shoulder Press

In a seated position, hold a barbell just past shoulder width apart, level with your collarbone.

Lift the weight up by extending, not locking your elbows. Keep your back straight, and head forward, avoiding hyperextension. Do not press the weight up behind your neck.

Spotters can be positioned on both sides of the bar or in front of you.

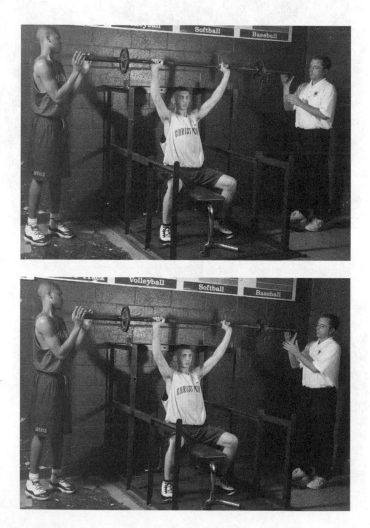

# Curls

In a seated position, hold a dumbbell in one hand. Place the non-exercising hand on the same knee. Place the elbow of the exercising arm on the inside of the same thigh.

Curl the weight up by bending your elbow.

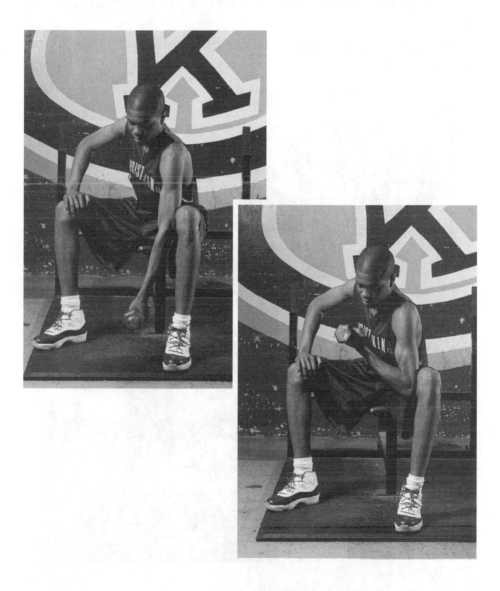

# Triceps

This exercise is also called a dumbbell kickback. Kneel with one knee on a bench. Bend at the waist and put the hand of the bent knee on the bench. With the opposite hand, lift the weight to chest height so it is parallel to the floor. Bending your elbow to a 90-degree angle, extend it backwards, making sure not to lock it.

If available, a weight machine is much more effective for triceps exercises.

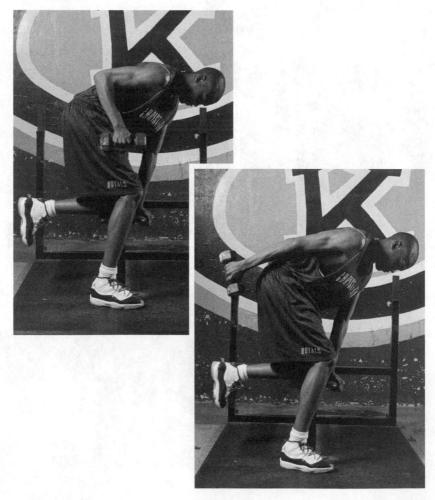

# Hang Cleans

This is a multi-joint exercise for power. Place the barbell on a rack or two platforms at shin level. Grip the bar just past shoulder width apart. Stand with your shins a few inches from the bar, with your knees and hips flexed and your shoulders resting over the bar.

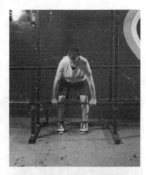

In one explosive motion, rise up on your toes while extending your knees and hips. Do not lift the weight up with your back. At the same time, shrug your shoulders to lift the weight.

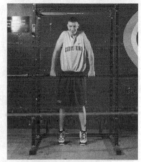

At the highest point on your toes, flex your elbows and bring the bar to shoulder height, making sure to keep your elbows pointing forward.

From this position, lower your body slightly, but do not let your knees go beyond your feet.

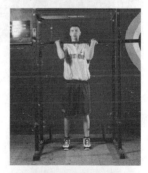

Rise and repeat the process.

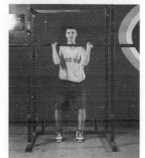

# Clean and Press

This exercise is performed in the same manner as the hang clean, except that the bar is lifted over the head.

In one motion, extend your legs and press the bar over head.

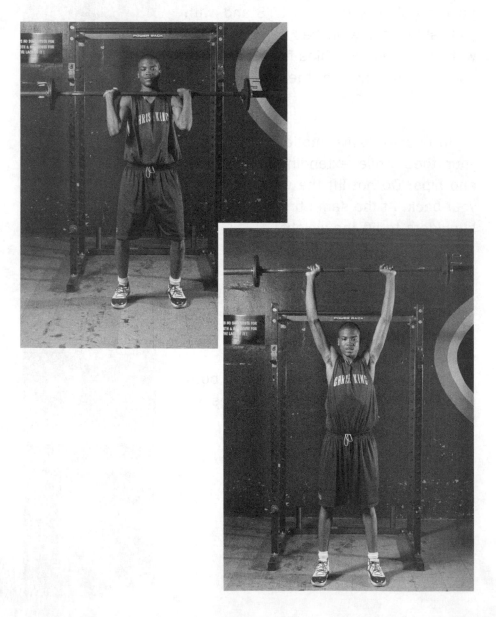

# Dead Lift

Stand over the bar with your hands just past shoulder width apart, shins close to the bar, shoulders over the bar, knees and hips flexed, and head forward. Grip the bar with one hand over the bar and one hand under the bar.

In one motion, extend your knees and hips, raising the bar. Keep your back straight, making sure not to lift the bar with your back.

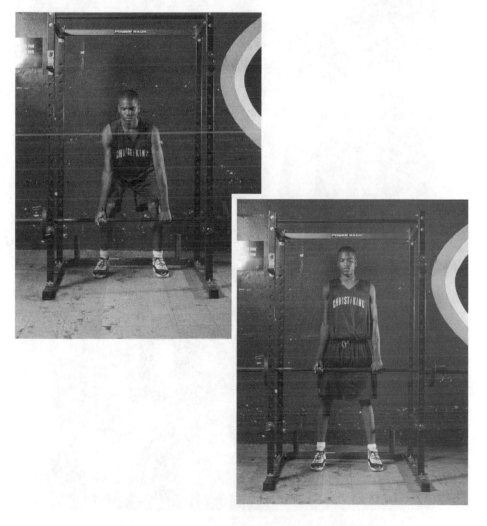

# Wrist Curls

Sit on a bench with the tops of your forearms resting on your thighs. Hold the bar with your palms facing forward and curl the weight up.

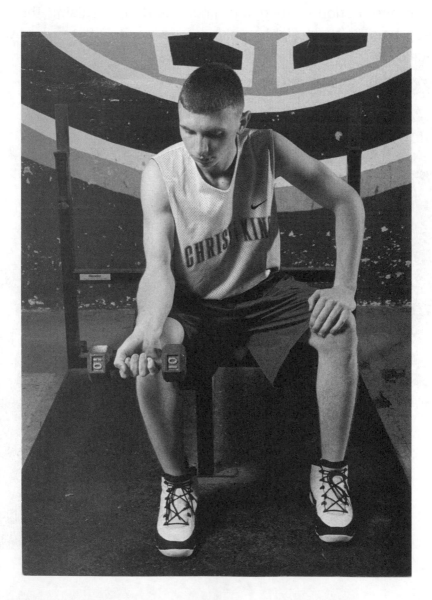

# Abdominal Exercises

Lie on your back with your knees bent and your hands resting behind your head.

Lift your shoulders off the floor, bringing your face toward the ceiling. Do not jerk your head forward or pull with your arms.

Make sure to breathe, and return to the starting position.

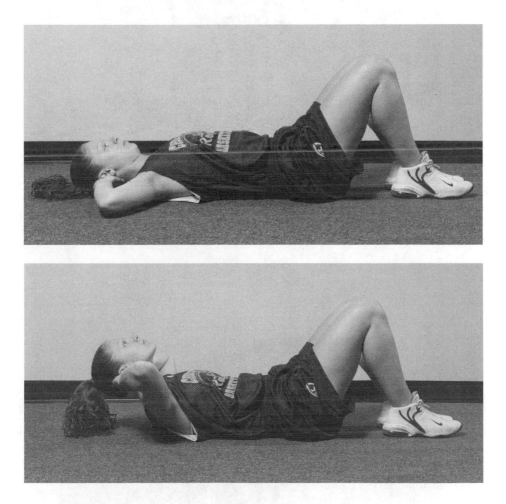

# Back Extension

Lie on your stomach on an exercise ball with your hands behind your head. Secure your feet to prevent slipping. Start with the trunk flexed, and slowly extend your back carefully to avoid hyperextension.

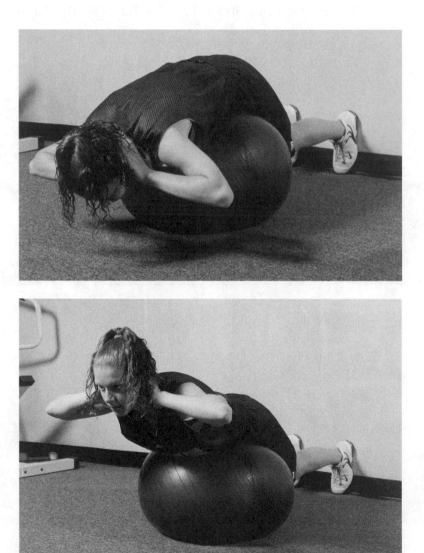

## Weight Lifting Exercises: Weight Machines

The exercises on the following pages make use of the weight machines you'll find in most schools. Just as when you're using free weights, form is important on weight machines, too.

# Leg Press

Sit in the leg press seat with your legs bent to approximately a 45-degree angle.

Slowly extend your legs, but do not lock your knees.

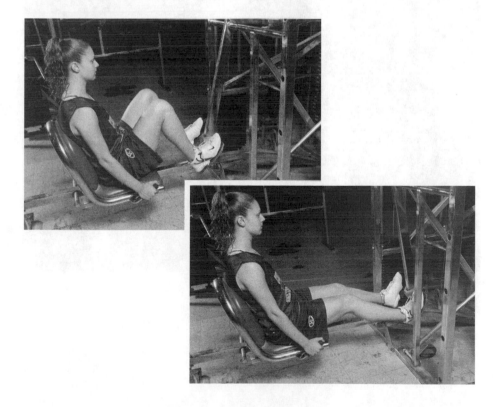

# Heel Raises

While sitting in the leg press seat, extend your legs, but do not lock the knees.

Push forward with your toes.

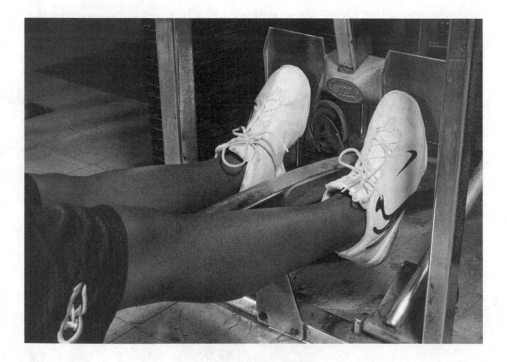

# Leg Curls

Lie on your stomach on the leg curl bench. If the bench is flat, place a folded towel under your hips to avoid hyper-extending the back.

Place your feet under the pads, trying to avoid excessive external rotation. Curl the weight up, but don't lift your hips off the bench or arch your back.

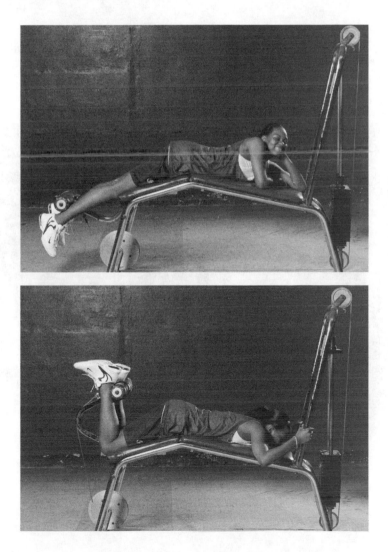

# Bench Press

Lie flat on the bench with your feet on the bench and position yourself so the bar is close to your chest.

Extend your arms upward, making sure not to lock the elbows.

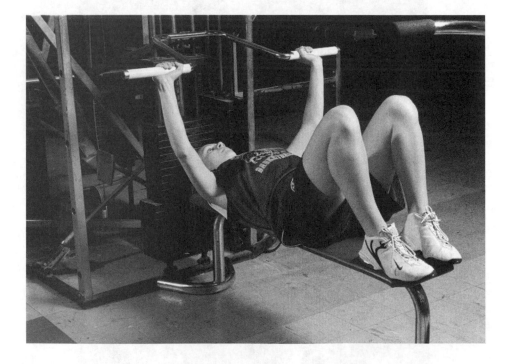

# Lat Pull-Downs

Reach up and grip the bar further than shoulder with apart.

Pulling the bar down to your collarbone, "chicken wing" your arms so that the triceps are to either side of your trunk.

Contrary to popular belief, do not bring the bar behind your neck as this can cause neck and shoulder strain.

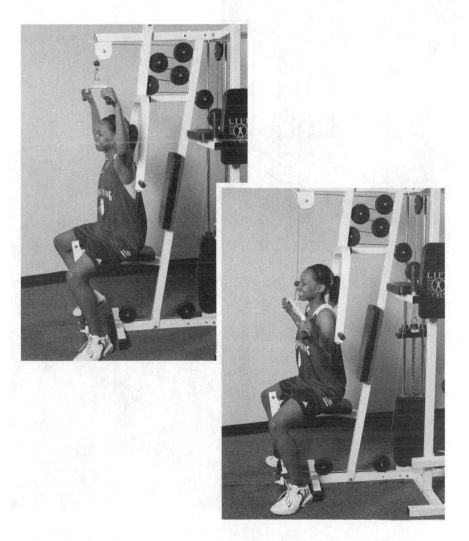

# Forward Shoulder Press

In a seated position, face the machine with the bar positioned in front of your shoulders.

Extend your arms forward and up, but do not lock the elbows.

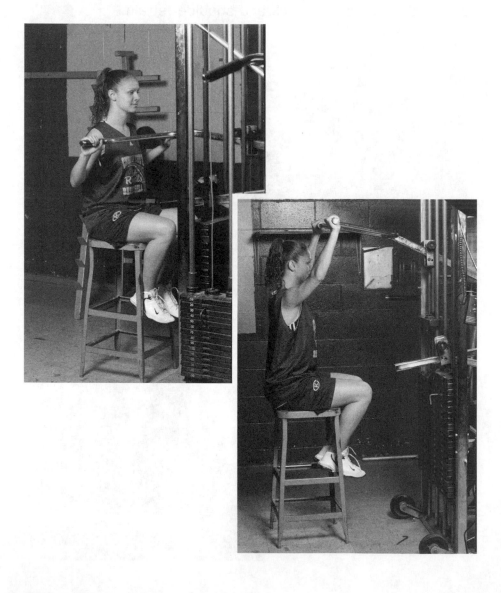

# Curls

With your back straight and arms extended, grip the bar while standing close to the machine. This decreases the inclination to arch your back.

Curl the bar up, but do not arch your back.

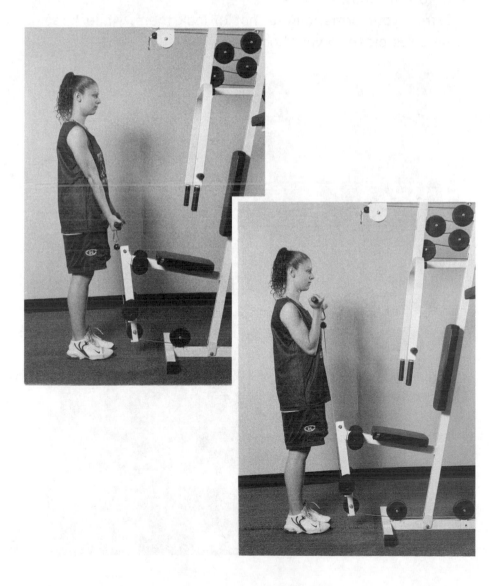

# Triceps

For this exercise, use the lat pull down bar or triceps extension attachment.

Standing close to the machine, place your hands over the top of the bar, making sure that your elbows are bent and are close to your body.

Extend your arms, careful not to lock them, while keeping your elbows close to your body.

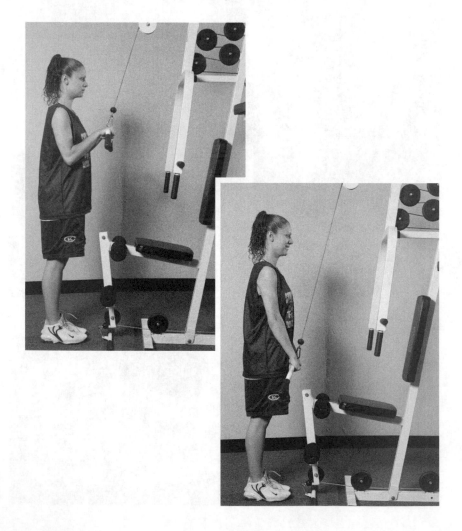

# Chapter 7

# Principles of Endurance Training

**D**uring the course of a basketball game it's normal for a player to run nearly two miles. Although the action is stop and go, making cardiovascular endurance of smaller initial importance when compared to other basketball skills, there are many benefits you will receive from an endurance training program. Endurance training, or aerobic exercise, improves the efficiency of the heart and lungs, which supply oxygen to exercising muscles. Because endurance training allows you to perform more work with less effort, you will be able to recover more quickly from exercise, be better prepared for higher intensity exercises, and more efficiently decrease weight and body fat.

## Applications of Endurance Training

Running, cycling, step machines, swimming, and aerobic classes are all forms of endurance training. These activities are a good alternative or supplement to traditional training exercises since they provide aerobic benefits and help to develop coordination. For endurance training to be effective, exercise must

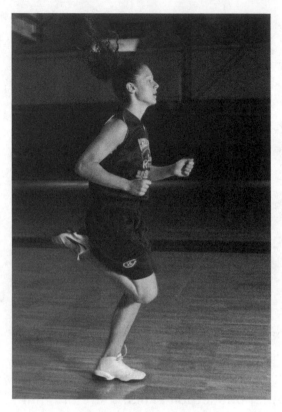

be continuous for at least twenty minutes.

Fitness circuits are another great option—if your town does not have a nature trail, your coach can help you develop an appropriate circuit. A sample trail could consist of calisthenics (e.g., push-ups, sit-ups, leg lifts, jumping jacks, wall jumps), interspersed with endurance runs. Players are typically broken down into small groups located in each corner of a gym. After 2 to 3 laps around the gym for a warm-up, each group stops at each corner to perform the pre-determined calisthenics for that corner. This is only one option; any type of cross training or alternate activities mixed into training will keep the body and mind fresh.

Here are some tips to keep in mind when conducting endurance training:

- Warm up, cool down, and stretch before and after each session.
- Wear appropriate foot gear. Basketball players are attached to their shoes, but unfortunately, basketball shoes aren't made for prolonged endurance runs. For long training runs, consider an appropriate running shoe. For step machines or cycling, however, basketball sneakers are fine.
- When running, try to stay on softer surfaces such as tracks or asphalt. If you choose to cross-train to mix up your work-

out every few days, try and avoid bumpy or irregular surfaces that can cause ankle or knee injuries.

- An average of 3 to 5 days per week of endurance training
  will develop your cardiovascular system as well as shed
  unwanted pounds and fat.
- Continuous activity for 20 to 30 minutes and not more than
  45 minutes is adequate. This is especially important when
  it comes to running due to the fact that a higher risk of
  injury occurs as time and distances increase.

There are two ways to maintain a pace that will allow you to
gain aerobic benefits. The simplest form is the "talk" pace, which
means that you should easily be able to converse while working
out without losing your breath. The preferred method, however, is
to establish your target heart rate, or the ideal amount of beats
per minute. By doing the following simple calculation you can
establish your personal target heart rate by which to judge your
aerobic activity. For a correct number, locate either the carotid
artery in the neck, or the radial artery in the wrist. To determine
your target heart rate, use this formula:

**220 – your age = max heart rate**
**Max heart rate x 60 percent = lower end of your target heart rate**
**Max heart rate x 80 percent = upper end of your target heart rate**

**Example using a 15-year-old player:**
**220 – 15 = 205.**
**205 x 60% = 123**
**205 x 80% = 164**

Using this formula, a 15-year-old player will have a target
heart rate in the range of 123 and 164 beats per minute.
Anything below the minimum will have little affect on

endurance capabilities. On the other hand, anything above the maximum can be dangerous.

# Application of Target Heart Rate

Begin your chosen activity at a comfortable pace. After 2 minutes check your pulse. You should count the number of beats for 15 seconds and multiply that number by 4. You will then see where the number is in relation to your previously established target heart rate. If the number is too low, you will need to increase the pace. If it's too high, you should slow down. If you have low endurance or are just starting out, begin the program at the lower end of your target heart rate and gradually progress from there.

Increase the intensity and duration by no more than 10 percent per week. This will aid in preventing injuries and staleness.

# Supplemental Training

At 1 to 2 times per week include Fartlek type training in your workout. Fartlek training is a series of continuous endurance activities that vary in speed. You can apply this on a road, for example, by running for 5 minutes at a steady pace and then increasing the speed, but not sprinting, for the distance between 2 telephone poles. Run another 5 minutes and then increase the pace between 3 telephone poles. Continue in a similar fashion for at least 20 to 30 minutes. This training can also be performed on a bike or step machine by manually increasing your speed or by choosing an interval program. The time interval for the speed increase is up to you, but should be in the range of 15 to 60 seconds.

# Chapter 8

# Speed Training

**Y**our teammate has pulled down a great rebound and you're sprinting down court looking for the outlet pass, but your opponent is right on your heels. In situations like this, the faster player will get the pass.

Great plays in basketball are made and broken by speed, and speed development is just as important for basketball players as it is for sprinters. This is one of the reasons that many coaches "recommend" that their players join the track team. Yet running and running fast, however similar, are two separate skills that must be honed using different methods.

Unlike endurance training, speed training is considered anaerobic because the short bursts of energy do not use oxygen but glycogen and creatine stored in the muscles. Due to the limited supply of oxygen available to sustain the high level of intensity on the muscles, lactic acid levels increase in the muscles, creating fatigue. This is why you can only run a limited distance at high intensity before your legs become heavy and tired.

**Most coaches agree that there is no perfect style of running. However, there is a general consensus among coaches that running requires basic style criteria including:**

- Push off the ground with force.
- Stay on your toes to accelerate.
- Legs should drive forward by lifting the drive leg so the thigh is nearly parallel to the ground. Your heel should be nearly on the buttocks, prepared to swing through to the next stride, which track coaches call turn over.
- Your arms should be relaxed and bent to about a 90-degree angle.
- When running, your arms can swing forward and back, but shouldn't go higher than your shoulders or behind your trunk on the back swing. Running with your arms swinging across the front of your body wastes energy and can cause strain on your back.

*Continued on next page* →

We've already discussed how basketball is a multi-directional sport that requires you to move quickly going forward, backward, laterally, diagonally, and side-to-side. To develop these skills, you must combine strength, agility, and running drills into your training sessions.

Running quickly requires coordinated movements of the arms and legs in an efficient and powerful stride. During adolescence, drills which aid coordination are especially important, due to the relative awkwardness of the age. Although athletes inherently know how to run, training to be a more efficient runner will help the athlete beat out the competition and get to the ball faster. Development of these skills could mean the difference between a win and a loss.

- Keep your hands relaxed and slightly cupped. Running with a fist wastes energy and could limit your reactions to the ball.
- Keep your head and trunk straight. Leaning too far forward can cause lower back fatigue and injury.
- Keep the muscles in your face relaxed.
- Talking about speed means talking about the ability both to run quickly *and* react quickly. In the fast-paced game of basketball, players must respond to opponents covering them and also to the flight path of the ball. Developing fast reaction time will help make you a more successful player, and may also limit mental mistakes. Fine-tuning this skill can be accomplished only through training and sport-specific drills. Good physical condition and rest breaks will help you defend against the effects of fatigue on your reaction time. When you are tired, the skills you learn through the speed drills will pay off. ■

# Applying Speed Training

- Warm up, cool down, and stretch before and after each session.
- Depending on the time of season, speed training will be conducted either 2 or 3 days per week. The higher the intensity, the more time will be required between days.
- Alternate between "hard" workout days and easy ones.

The majority of speed repetitions should be under 60 seconds. Markings such as baselines, foul lines, and the mid-court line can be used as repetition landmarks.

Depending on the program guidelines, intensity can range from a half speed stride to an all-out sprint. Remember, not every speed session needs to be done at top speed. Avoid increasing intensity and duration by more than 10 percent per week.

## Form Drills

These drills can be performed following the general warm up and stretch session. They are designed to develop the previously described running techniques by focusing on specific body parts. The form drill should be performed using the full length of the court.

# High Knees

As you run, swing your arms, relax your hands, and lift your knees high so your thighs are parallel to the ground.

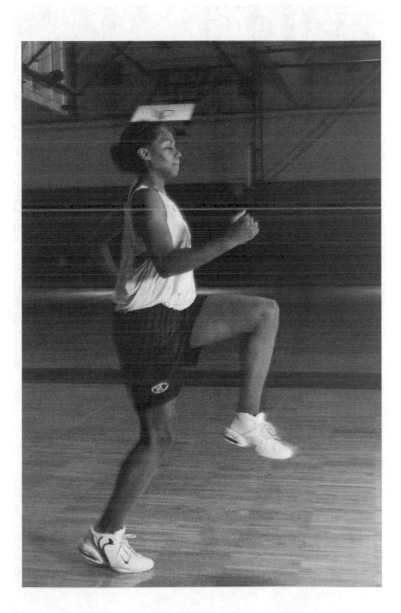

# Butt Kicks

Swing your arms and relax your hands as you run, kicking your heels into your buttocks. Your thighs should be facing forward.

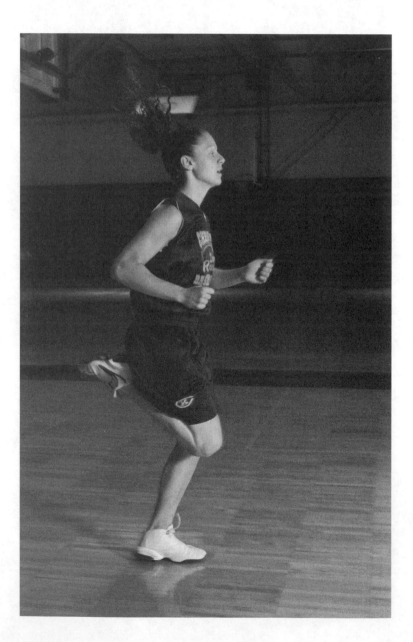

# Toe-Pulls

Mimic a pair of scissors as you run, pulling your toes back when your foot leaves the ground and pushing your toes forward as your foot approaches the ground. Be sure to swing your arms and relax your hands.

# Carioca

Stand facing the right sideline. In a side step motion, cross your left leg behind your right leg and side step. Then, cross your left leg in front of your right leg and as your leg crosses in front of your other leg, "pop" up your knee in a quick motion. After going down the court to the far baseline, move to the starting baseline and work the other leg.

# Backward Run

Run backward emphasizing arm and leg movement.

# Lunges

Keep your back and head straight, and with your eyes forward, take a step with your right leg. Your knee should be bent to about a 90-degree angle and should not extend beyond your foot. Swing your left leg through by raising on the toes of your right foot, and bend your left leg so that your heel is close to your buttocks. Then, swing your left leg through to the lunge position. Alternate legs as you move down court.

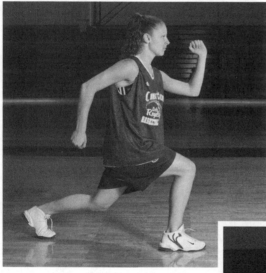

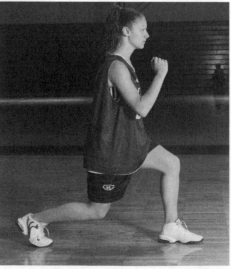

# Sprint Regimens

Essentially, the basketball court is broken down into functional training grids comprised of the baselines, foul lines, sidelines, and the mid-court line. The average basketball court is between 84 and 94 feet by 50 feet wide and the distance to the foul line is 19 feet from the baseline. You and your coach can use these landmarks to establish speed-training distances.

The speed programs described later in this book incorporate running drills that stretch from baseline to the opposite foul line and avoid sprinting baseline to baseline since space is needed to decelerate. The traditional "suicides" are also an option—these drills include running from baseline to foul line, back to baseline, mid court back to baseline, and then far foul line to baseline. Depending on intensity, this can be done for various repetitions. This form of workout will emphasize the anaerobic energy system.

## Reaction Time Drills

The effectiveness of these drills is dependent on the quickness of response. Many of the drills described later in the Vision Training Chapter will also enhance reaction time.

# Quick Feet Response

For this drill you will be positioned with your knees bent, feet quickly "chopping," hands in front of you in the "ready" position, head straight, and eyes forward. Your coach should be in plain view. On the whistle, quickly respond by angling your body in the direction the coach points. Make sure that your feet are still "chopping" when you respond. Directions commonly given from the coach are forward, to the right or the left, and move forward or back three steps.

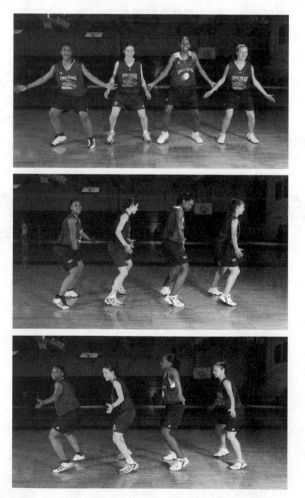

# Mirror Drill

For this drill, two players stand facing each other. One player puts their hands up and quickly moves them to different positions. The partner responds by mirroring the actions.

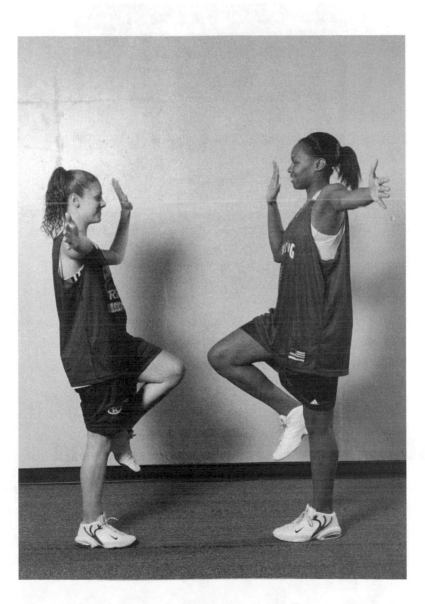

# Blind Response

Lie on your back with your feet on the baseline. The coach will bounce a ball a few feet in front of you. When you hear the ball hit the floor, get up and retrieve the ball as quickly as possible.

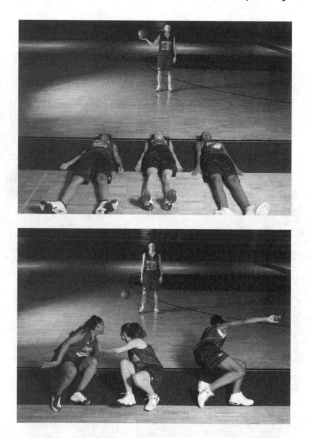

# Blind Response Standing

Stand on the baseline with your back to the court, while moving your feet in a chopping motion. The coach will bounce a ball no farther than to the distance of the foul line. When you hear the ball bounce, quickly turn around and retrieve the ball.

# Chapter 9

# Power Training

**S**trength is an important contributor to athletic success and injury prevention. True athletic success is achieved when your newly developed strength can be called upon to respond quickly and forcefully in the shortest time possible. When you have achieved this, you have not only strength, but power as well.

Power exerted by your muscles allows you to accelerate down the court, jump high to block a shot, or even make a dunk. Power is developed through a combination of strength training to increase the amount of force your muscles can exert combined with training your neuromuscular system to take this strength and unleash it quickly. Despite the neuro-physiological complexity of the mechanisms involved in developing power, the actual methods to develop power are quite simple.

Transfer training, also known as plyometrics, will unleash the strength gained during your strength-training program. This type of training involves rapidly putting your muscles in a pre-stretch position and then quickly jumping or throwing. The process is repeated for a specified number of repetitions.

Plyometrics uses the muscle's natural elastic properties to achieve a rapid stretch position where the muscle spindle is excited. This results in the Myotatic Stretch Reflex, which is a reactive muscle contraction that augments the developing muscle's ability to forcefully and rapidly contract at a higher level. With a weight-training program that includes plyometrics, you will achieve new heights and speeds.

# Applying Power Training

Before you begin this power drill program, you should have no less than 6 weeks of strength training to prepare your muscles for high intensity work.

Here are some quick facts to get you started with power training:

- Power drills should be done no more than twice per week with 48 to 72 hours rest between sessions. The power drills are to be conducted no more than 4 weeks during the preseason phase of your conditioning program and should be done on lifting days.
- Start with 1 set of 5 repetitions for 1 to 2 weeks to allow your body to adjust to the stress. After the adjustment stage, you can average 3 sets of 6 repetitions, but do not do more than 10 repetitions per set.
- Start with low impact drills and progress to higher impact activities, making sure that you follow all safety guidelines. These drills are intended for preseason workouts and should be done before weight training and sprint/speed drills and after skill work. As always, be sure to warm up, cool down, and stretch before and after each training session.

## POWER TRAINING SAFETY

Many power drills may be stressful to your body. Prepare for this workout gradually, follow the recommended form, and stop exercising if pain or injury occur.

Athletes younger than 12 years should not perform jumps from heights or a high numbers of sets and repetitions.

When doing depth jumps, start with heights of 18 inches, progressing no higher than 24 inches.

Avoid jumping directly onto the basketball court for depth jumps. Instead, jump onto wrestling or gymnastic mats to decrease the shock to your body.

Prior to doing any power drills you should be able to do at least 10 push-ups and squat your body weight.

Avoid power drills if you are injured or fatigued.

Use proper technique at all times.

Jump boxes should have a non-skid bottom to prevent sliding. The tops of the boxes should be padded as well to prevent injuries.

Young athletes should not use any form of external resistance when doing these drills. This includes ankle weights or weights on the shoulders.

# Lower Extremities

The following drills are intended to increase your vertical and horizontal power capabilities. They will improve your ability to jump for a shot, block, or dunk, as well as pass or complete a lay up.

# Wall Taps

Wall taps emphasize vertical explosiveness.

Stand facing the wall, with your feet shoulder width apart and your arms extended upward. Keep your back straight.

Bend your knees slightly and jump off the ground, emphasizing pushing off with your ankles and toes.

Reach high up on the wall while maintaining this form. As soon as your toes hit the ground, immediately repeat the process. Your heels should not touch the ground.

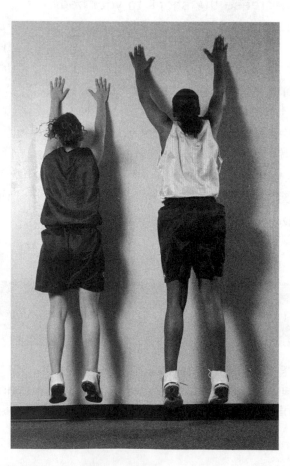

# Squat Jumps

Squat jumps emphasize vertical explosiveness.

Start in a squatting position, keeping your feet shoulder width apart. Your thighs should be parallel to the ground and your shoulders over your knees.

Swing your arms up and extend your ankles and knees, reaching up with your arms.

As soon as your toes hit the ground, resume the squat position and jump again.

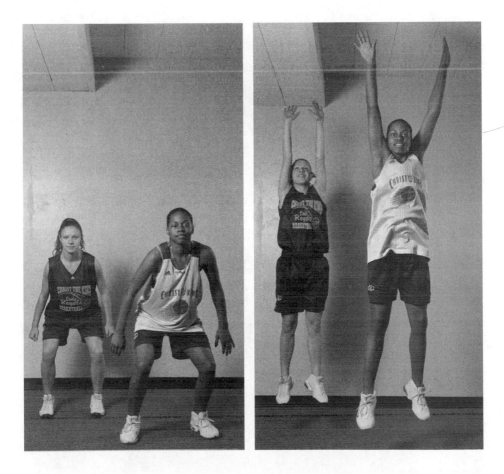

# Double-Leg Tuck Jumps

Double leg tuck jumps emphasize vertical explosiveness.

From a squatting position with your feet shoulder width apart, thighs parallel to the ground, and your shoulders over your knees, swing your arms, extend your ankles and knees, and reach up with your arms.

When you are in the air, flex your hips and bring your heels to your buttocks.

As soon as your toes hit the ground, resume the squatting position and repeat the jump sequence.

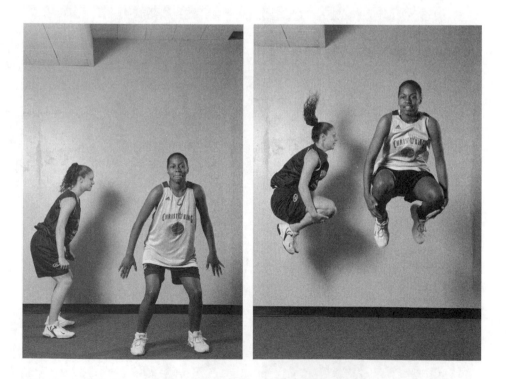

# Depth Jumps

Depth jumps emphasize vertical explosiveness.

Stand on a box that is at least 18 inches and is no higher than 24 inches.

Step off the box with both feet and then flex your hips and knees into a semi-squat position with your feet shoulder width apart and your shoulders over your knees. After landing from the jump, quickly extend your ankles, knees, and hips into a vertical jump, while reaching overhead with your arms.

After landing from the jump, repeat the sequence.

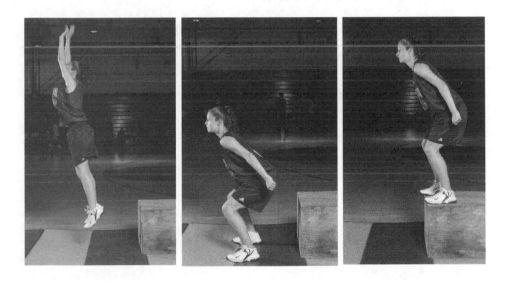

# Box Hops

Box hops emphasize vertical and horizontal explosiveness.

Arrange 4 to 5 boxes, each 18 to 24 inches high, 3 to 4 feet apart in a straight line.

Hop over the boxes with a double leg tuck jump.

As soon as your feet hit the ground, rapidly jump over the next box, avoiding a stutter step or double hop between boxes.

After you jump over the last box, sprint back to the beginning and resume the sequence.

# Power Bounds

Power bounds emphasize horizontal explosiveness.

A power bound is basically an over stride where your feet bounce off the floor.

The thigh of your lead leg should be parallel to the ground, while your back leg is flexed.

Swing your arms to aid in the momentum of the bound.

# Repeat Forward Hops

Repeat Forward Hops emphasize horizontal explosiveness. Focus on jumping forward, not up, during this drill.

From a squatting position with your feet shoulder width apart, thighs parallel to the ground, and your shoulders over your knees, swing your arms and jump forward, flexing your hips, bringing your heels to your buttocks, and reaching forward with you feet and arms.

As soon as your feet hit the ground, repeat the sequence.

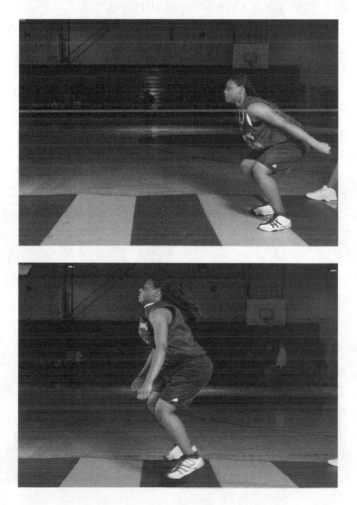

## Upper Extremities

The following drills are designed to develop your upper body power, helping you send crisp chest and bounce passes, as well as increasing your strength to receive passes.

# Wall Push-Up Claps

Stand approximately 2 feet from the wall and place your hands on the wall, just past shoulder width apart.

Keeping your head, back, and hips straight, bend your elbows and move toward the wall.

Forcefully push away from the wall, and clap your hands.

After clapping your hands once, drop toward the wall, absorbing the shock by bending your elbows.

Rapidly repeat the sequence.

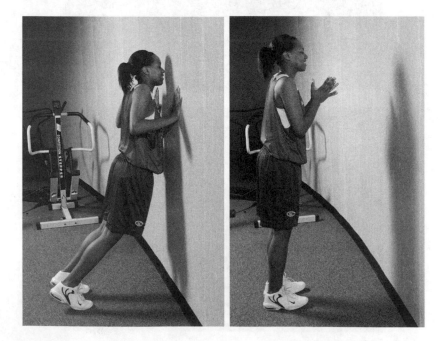

# Modified Push-Up Claps

Place your knees and hands on the floor, making sure to keep your head, back, and hips straight.

Bring your body to the floor by bending your elbows.

Lift off the floor by extending your elbows and clap your hands once while in the air.

When returning to the floor, make sure to bend your elbows to absorb the excess shock.

Rapidly repeat the sequence.

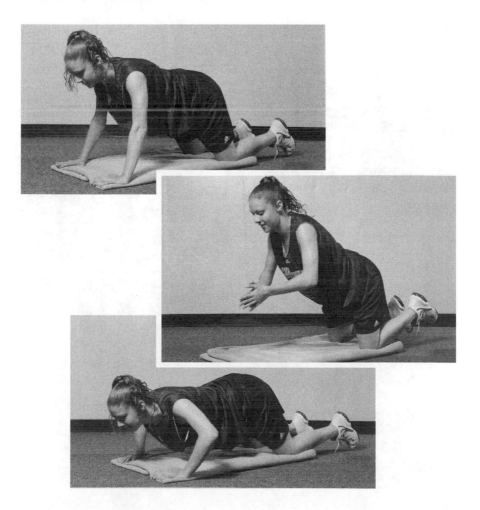

# Regular Push-Up Claps

In a push-up position, making sure to keep your head, back, hips, and knees straight.

Bring your body to the floor by bending your elbows.

Lift off the floor by extending your elbows and clap your hands once while in the air.

When returning to the floor, make sure to bend your elbows to absorb the excess shock.

Rapidly repeat the sequence.

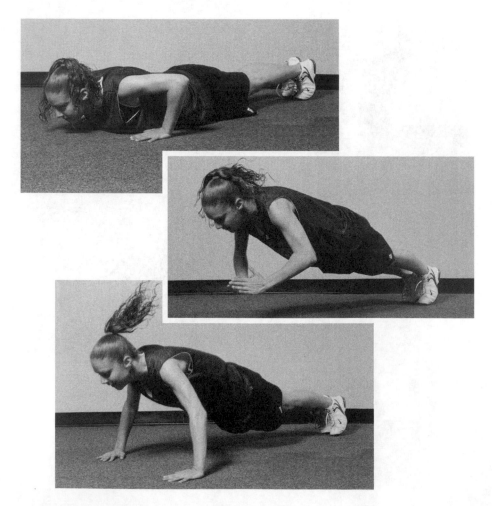

# Medicine Ball Pass

For this drill, two athletes stand facing each other 8 to 10 feet apart.

With either a weighted basketball or medicine ball, one player will make a chest pass to their partner, who will bring the ball into their chest. It is important to flex your arms when you catch the ball to absorb the shock.

As soon as you catch the ball, quickly pass it back to your partner. Rapidly repeat the sequence.

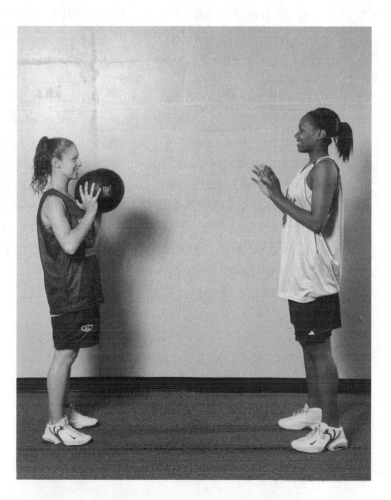

# POWER SHOES

Recently, power shoes have gained popularity, with manufacturers claiming that the shoes stretch and contract the calf muscles more effectively, therefore building the muscle by allowing the heel to drop behind the fore foot platform. Essentially, the shoes replicate the Myotatic Stretch Reflex Principle.

Keep in mind, though, that research concludes that power can be gained just as effectively through a combination of strength training and power drills. Athletes need to be cautious when wearing these shoes because their height and lack of stability may increase the risk of ankle sprains, strains, and tendonitis.

Although power shoes may take the credit for increasing the height of your jumps, keep in mind that a vertical jump involves more than the calf muscles. Vertical jumping is a multi-joint activity that incorporates the calves, quadriceps, hamstrings, buttocks, back and arms. These muscles should be trained as a unit to hone this specific skill. My recommendation is that if you opt to use power shoes, use them cautiously and sparingly as an adjunct to a comprehensive plyometric program.

# Chapter 10
# Vision Training

In literature, eyes are known as windows to the soul, but in basketball, eyes can be the doorway to success. Visual acuity, peripheral vision, and depth perception all play a role in basketball success by helping you locate the ball as well as providing sensory information about where the ball and players are at any given time. We've all heard coaches say, "Keep your eye on the ball!" and indeed developing this skill will help you be a better player.

Like the cardiovascular, respiratory, and muscular systems, training of the eyes must be included in any conditioning program. Vision training is inexpensive and requires little time to realize results.

Although everyone can benefit from vision training, this program will particularly help athletes who have poor hand-eye coordination, bad timing in positioning, excessive eye rubbing, squinting, an increased injury rate, poor balance, and inconsistent performance. Many times the initiation of vision training reveals a need for prescription glasses or contact lenses, as was the case for Charlie Sheen's character in the baseball movie *Major League,* who had incredible pitching talent, but poor accuracy because he couldn't see properly.

When you visit an eye doctor or optometrist to determine whether your vision needs correction, the exam will make use of both a traditional eye chart as well as more sophisticated methods for evaluating eyesight The doctor will also measure binocular vision, depth perception, reaction time, eye teaming, and focusing ability, as well as hand-eye coordination, reaction time and visual speed and accuracy.

Even if you think your vision is perfect (many doctors consider both 20/20 and 20/40 to be acceptable) keep in mind that headaches are a good indicator of eye stress.

If you're one of the lucky ones whose vision is problem-free, vision training can still be of enormous use to improve dynamic visual acuity, depth perception, and peripheral vision. Dynamic visual acuity refers to the eye's ability to focus on a moving object, and can decrease with eye fatigue. Depth perception relates to how the eyes focus and fixate on an object. It allows you to gauge the arc and effort needed to make a shot given a certain distance, as well as judging other players' positions. Consistent over or under shooting may be an indication of a problem with depth perception. Peripheral vision refers to the ability to see laterally, ideally 180 degrees. It is said that New York Knicks legend Bill Bradley had 195-degree peripheral vision; talk about eyes in the back of the head!

## Applying Vision Training

The following exercises can be conducted at home, requiring little time and equipment. Try to complete the exercises daily. Each exercise requires only 3 sets of 10 to 15 repetitions. Unlike weight training, there are no intensity limits to vision training. Focus visually and mentally on the object and tasks at hand.

# Visual Acuity Exercise A

Hold a pencil in front of your face at arm's length.

Bring the pencil slowly toward your nose, focusing on the pencil until you see 2 images of it. Bring the pencil back to arm's length and repeat the process.

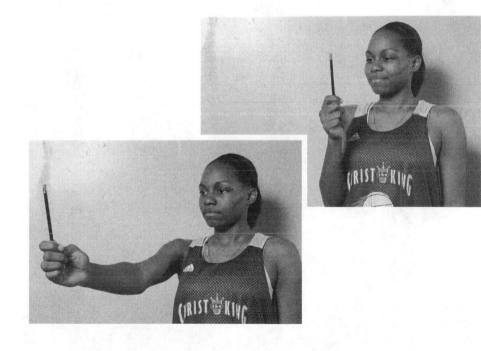

# Visual Acuity Exercise B

Tape or paint 4 colored squares on a basketball. Two players will pass the ball back and forth, concentrating on seeing 1 color at a time.

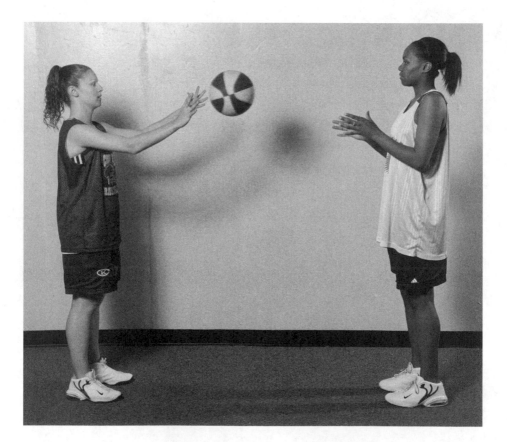

# Depth Perception

Hold a pencil near your nose (without seeing double) and another at arm's length.

Alternate positions of the pencils, moving them farther away from and closer to your face.

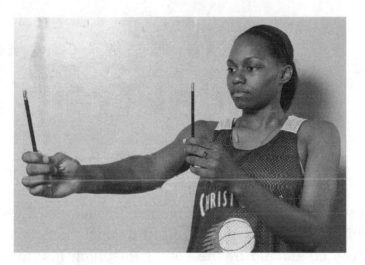

# Peripheral Vision

Have a partner stand behind you while you are looking forward. Your partner will move to either side of you, holding up a number of fingers. Identify the number of fingers held up as soon as they appear to you.

# Chapter 11

# Mental Training

Sports psychology plays an integral role in preparing elite and professional athletes for competition. For example, the success gained by professional and Olympic athletes using mental imagery has been supported by documented research. One study conducted by the Lerner Research Institute of the Cleveland Clinic Foundation found that people who just thought about bending their elbow for 15 minutes 5 times per week increased their strength 13.5 percent, without ever lifting a weight. Try experimenting with vertical jump thoughts or making the game winning shot.

Although less frequently used at lower levels, the high school basketball player is a prime candidate to take advantage of sports psychology principles. Pressures and stress from family, friends, life, and sports can wreak havoc on an athlete's play and health. Distractions, motivation, burnout, lack of rest, improper diet, and psyching techniques are all mental factors that come into play for the high school basketball player, but are rarely addressed at this level. Despite a well-planned physical and tactical program, an athlete will not reach his or her full potential unless the mind is trained as well as the body.

Mental imagery, which blends what the athlete has observed, been taught, and should do in a given situation, has been used by athletes, with great success. Think of mental imagery as running a video through your mind over and over, breaking the skills down to the smallest details, then watching and feeling yourself perform the skill in your mind. These parameters are then repeated in order to prepare the subconscious mind to execute the skill when physically required.

Young athletes sometimes have difficulty comprehending how the mind fuels the body. When you're taught a new skill, it eventually becomes a learned response through practice and repetition. Mental imagery can help you bring these learned responses to the forefront of your mind, allowing an automatic and smooth transition to superior performance. If you observe players on the free throw line you see how some hold up the ball, aligning it with the basket. What they may also be doing is running a video through their mind: recalling the ideal body mechanics, the flight of the ball, and visualizing the ball going into the net. Surprisingly, this can be done in the brief moments on the foul line; you just have to learn to train your brain.

# Technique

There are various ways to apply mental imagery. The key to success is total concentration. Some athletes choose a quiet room, others may choose rhythmical music in head phones, some like to lay down, others like to sit up. Coaches may choose to have players perform mental imagery on the bus to a game, or to arrive early for a game and have the players sit in the locker room. Mental imagery can be a short exercise while standing on the foul line, or can last for 15 minutes or more. In either scenario, you will get the most effectiveness from the exercise if you keep your eyes closed and allow yourself to concentrate. Like all skills, the more often you practice, the more proficient you will become.

**Here are some ideas to help you through a mental imagery exercise:**

- Hold a basketball while doing an exercise to relate the feel of the ball on your hand to your mind.

- Watch videos of yourself or of an accomplished player executing the skills you wish to do. If you are analyzing past performances or a newly learned skill, critique and correct, but try not to criticize. Stay positive.

- Hang up pictures, not only to admire, but also to analyze.

- Emphasize a sense of confidence. Adopt an "I can do it" attitude.

- Stay relaxed and breathe smoothly.

- Break skills down in segments. For example, consider a free throw (Your coach can make a brief outline for you on how a skill should be broken down):
    - Your eyes are focused on the basket.
    - Feel and see the ball in your hand and your feet on the floor.
    - Your ankles, knees, and shooting elbow are bending to prepare for the shot as it is stabilized by your hand.

- Rising on your toes, straightening your legs, and lifting your shooting hand towards the basket, feel the ball rolling out of your hand, off of your fingers, your wrist bending down, and the ball arcing towards the basket.
- See the ball go in!

• When it comes to plays, visualize where and when you need to be at a certain point on the floor. Like teaching dance steps, draw mental lines on the floor and visualize where team mates are and where and when you need to move.

• In your mind, watch yourself and feel yourself doing the task.

• Stay relaxed and be confident.

# Chapter 12

# Overtraining

**P**reparing for and playing high school basketball is a fun yet grueling process. An average season runs from the end of November to early March, if you're lucky enough to make the playoffs. Combine this with off-season training and summer leagues and camps, and high school basketball can become a year-round endeavor. Finding the balance between enjoyment, development, and competition can be difficult for many players, coaches, and parents.

The signs and symptoms of over-training, when an athlete has given up physically and emotionally, are subtle. One study determined that the number of young athletes burned out on their sport was as high as 70 percent. All too often athletes give up a sport because "it's not fun anymore," but this source of burnout can be avoided if the coach and parents create an environment where the athlete continues to develop as well as enjoy the sport.

Athletes can also experience physical burnout from simply overworking the body. Often this is unintentional and may even result from the very best intentions. Be careful to sidestep this easily avoidable pitfall. The body responds to a physical bell curve, where certain levels of stress need to be applied in order to receive gains. As the top of the curve is approached, however, the body begins to send out warning signs. If the stress is continued, the body will begin to slide down the other side of the curve, where injury, illness, or emotional problems can occur.

# Causes of Burnout and Over-training

## Poor Program Design

Excessive emphasis on conditioning without adequate rest is detrimental. If proper rest and variety are not encouraged, players will not only become mentally and physically stagnant, but will "freelance" on their own, running the risk of injury. When developing conditioning programs, incorporate recovery days, and change the intensity or activity level during the year, utilizing periodization.

## Unrealistic Goals

Not every high school player has a future in the NBA. It is important to understand each

# Signs and Symptoms of Physical and Emotional Burnout

- Fatigue
- Slow recovery from workouts and injury
- Loss of appetite
- Sleep disturbances
- Apathy
- Irritability
- Depression
- Muscle soreness
- Muscle atrophy—decrease in the size and strength of a muscle
- Decreased neuromuscular function
- Increased resting heart rate, typically 5 to 10 beats above normal
- Increased blood pressure
- Increased susceptibility to flu-like symptoms

player's developmental, physical, and emotional abilities, and to push the athlete to reach for and achieve a goal that is challenging, yet attainable. Once one goal is attained, set more. Remember to include the athlete in your plans to gauge their commitment to achieving goals.

## Over Zealousness

Basketball coaches are notorious for being excitable, as are parents. Coaches should motivate the athletes, making sure not to degrade them.

## Psychosocial Pressure

Athletes should be given the opportunity to play without the pressures of the expectations of others.

## Poor Nutrition

Athletes need high-octane fuel to perform and prevent breakdown.

## Inadequate Rest

Encourage athletes to try to get 8 hours of sleep per night, and recognize when their bodies have had enough. Help athletes plan ahead if they will have to get up early for practice or stay late for a game.

# Care and Prevention of Burnout and Overtraining

To prevent physical and emotional burnout, remember the main causes and take care to avoid them. It's okay to be diligent with your workouts, but keep in mind that basketball season is long. Parents and coaches should be flexible with their athletes if they observe warning signs of over-training and allow ample time for recovery.

Coaches and parents should maintain an upbeat and motivating environment. Correct mistakes in a constructive fashion. Motivate athletes to perform in a positive manner, not through confrontation or indifference.

Know your athletes and push them, but not to the other side of the curve. Organize programs to stress athletic development, while incorporating rest and recovery.

Communicate with athletes and provide frequent feedback. If something needs to be improved, let the athlete know. A good way to do this, as well as motivate players, is to keep performance charts that measure improvements and slumps.

Encourage rest and nutrition. More isn't always better.

Teach or recommend relaxation techniques and stress management skills. It's no mistake that many colleges and professional teams have staff sport psychologists.

Finally, set realistic goals. Set the carrot in front of the athlete, but be sure they can grab it. When they can, set it out a little farther. Be patient. If goals aren't being achieved find out why first and then make an appropriate adjustment.

Chapter 13

# Game Day

**A**ll of your preparation culminates in the games you play throughout your high school basketball career. It can be a challenge for coaches and players to stay fresh and prepared for the 20 or so games per season. There are many factors that can influence an athlete on game day, from school, family, and social obligations to nutrition, rest, and preparation. Although some of these factors are unavoidable, it is up to you to create a game day routine that enhances your potential for success regardless of outside factors.

## Mental Preparation

To prepare for game day, your mind and body must be well rested. Therefore, game preparation actually starts the night before a game. Whatever your reason for normally staying up late—academics, social, or nerves—plan your time accordingly so that you get 8 hours of sleep on any night before a game.

Use the mental imagery techniques we discussed in the pre-

**164**

vious chapter and run a video through your mind of your play in the game. Do you have to mark up a certain player who has a particular skill you need to watch out for? Are you playing man to man or zone? Run that video in your mind to reflect your best performance or visualize a professional player and superimpose yourself over their skills. If you see yourself as successful, you will be successful.

Stay focused. Prior to the game distance yourself from all external distractions and concentrate on what you need to do during the game. All players differ in the amount of time they need to focus, but you should put aside at least 30 minutes prior to the coach's pre-game speech. During this time, some players like to dribble a ball, while others sit with a personal CD player listening to their own "psych music." Regardless of what you do, don't underestimate the value of mental preparation.

## Dietary Preparation

Like rest, dietary preparation begins the night before with a good dinner. The morning of a game, make sure to eat a healthy breakfast that may include any of the following: bagels, pancakes, waffles, oatmeal, non-frosted cereal, fruit, juice, or milk. For lunch, avoid fast foods such as hamburgers and hot dogs. An ideal lunch would include pasta, bread, and fruits. Coaches may be able to coordinate the best lunch with your school cafeteria. Depending on game time, you may or may not be able to eat dinner. If the game is after school, you probably will have time to eat only a snack of pretzels, crackers, or a sports bar. If game time is later, you will most likely have time to eat a dinner, which should be carbohydrate-based to supply quick energy. I recommend avoiding red meat or junk food for dinner. Regardless of what you eat, make sure you give yourself two hours to fully digest before game time.

Some athletes snack before the game or at half time. Though fruit is a good choice for snack food, some find that it upsets their stomach. Experiment with bananas and oranges during practice. The correct type and amount of food can make a great difference in how your body and mind perform during a game. You should never skip a meal on game day.

You may not realize it, but you can lose enough water through sweat to affect your performance during a game. To combat this, store up on about 10 glasses of water during the course of the day. At lunch and prior to the game, consume 12 to 16 ounces of a sports drink as well.

# Game Considerations

Although players and coaches understandably get caught up in the excitement during a game adhering to exercise physiology principles during the game can keep you competing at optimal performance levels. If your opponent does not consider these principles, this could even give you the edge to win the game.

Be sure to get a good warm-up and stretch prior to game time. Most teams have a specific routine they follow before a game, but try to include some of the suggested stretches in the Flexibility chapter to get your body and mind ready to compete.

Hydration remains a key consideration, as basketball players can lose over a quart of water in sweat per hour. With a loss of water as little as 2 percent of your body weight, muscle function can be affected, and higher rates of water loss can increase the risk of a heat related illness. To prevent this, drink 5 to 10 ounces of water or a sports drink every 15 minutes during the game. If the gym is uncomfortably warm, the coach should consider providing cool, wet towels for players to put over their heads when they come out of the game for a substitution or time-out. This can help dissipate heat as well as refresh an overheated player.

An idea that is growing in popularity is to have players ride stationary bicycles for a few minutes instead of directly sitting down when they come out of the game. When a player comes out and sits immediately down on the bench, the blood has a tendency to pool in the legs and the muscles can potentially shorten. By riding the bike for as little as 3 to 5 minutes the blood is re-circulated and the muscles will stay loose prior to getting back on the floor. This form of active rest has been found to eliminate lactic acid faster than sitting down, thereby providing quicker recovery between shifts on the floor. This technique can also be done in the locker room at half time.

## Post Game

Post-game exercise principles are rarely considered, especially after a loss. However, what you do after any workout can affect your next day's performance. This takes on particular relevance if your team is involved in a multi-day tournament. To ensure optimum performance the next day, stretch after the game to avoid stiffness, and replenish fluids and energy stores by drinking water or sport drinks as well as eating a high carbohydrate meal within an hour of the game's end.

# Chapter 14

# Injury Reconditioning

In his wildest dreams Dr. James Naismith, the creator of basketball, couldn't have foreseen where the game he developed over 100 years ago would have progressed in terms of participation, technical skill, and physical development. Equally, he couldn't have predicted how the contemporary aggressive nature of basketball creates inherent risk factors for participants in the sport. One report puts the number of basketball related injuries requiring medical care as high as 1.6 million cases annually. A 1998 study conducted by the American Academy of Orthopedic Surgeons found that basketball was the number one sport to send athletes to emergency rooms, with nearly 200,000 athletes injured per year.

In the event of injury, immediate and proper medical care is vital to prevent complications and delays in healing.

The following programs are designed to recondition common basketball injuries by focusing on specific muscle groups. However, I strongly recommend that you seek medical attention prior to performing these exercises to ensure a proper diagnosis. In time, the same conditioning exercises can be used for a full recovery.

## Exercises for Flexibility and Strength

The following exercises can also serve as valuable tools to prevent the occurrence and severity of injuries to the feet, ankles, and shins, knees, and thighs, lower back, shoulders, and wrists and hands. For instance, athletes who complain of "weak ankles" should be put on the ankle/shin program and not rely solely on being taped or braced. The exercises should be done in the sequences presented for each body part. If pain occurs, decrease the resistance. If you still feel pain, stop the exercise and seek medical advice.

For each body part, flexibility exercises are presented first, followed by strengthening exercises. Flexibility exercises are labeled **F**; strengthening exercises are labeled **S**.

# Arch Flex No. 1

Roll your foot back and forth on a ball 50 times to loosen the arch.

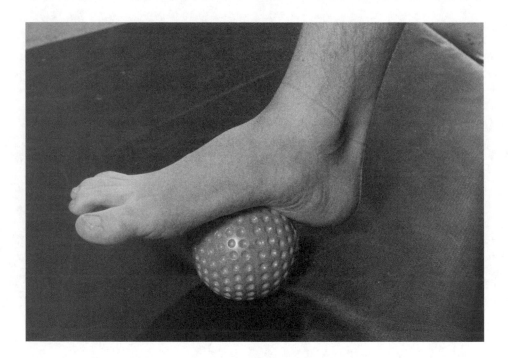

**ARCHES**

**F** = flexibility exercise
**S** = strengthening exercise

# Arch Flex No. 2

Pull your toes back. Hold the position for 15 seconds and repeat 3 to 5 times.

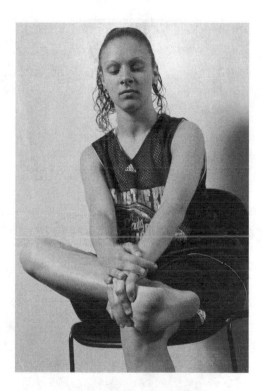

# Arch Flex No. 3

Stretch your calf and hold the position for 15 seconds. Repeat 3 to 5 times.

**ARCHES**

F = flexibility exercise
S = strengthening exercise

# Arch Strengthening No. 1

Crinkle a towel with your toes, with or without a weight as tolerated. Repeat 10 times.

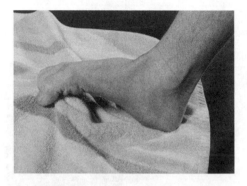

# Arch Strengthening No. 2

Pick up marbles with your toes. Repeat 50 times.

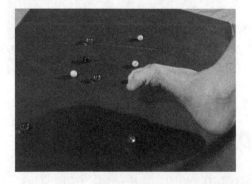

# S Arch Strengthening No. 3

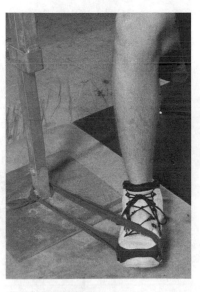

Perform the inversion exercise with a therapy band for 3 sets of 15. Only move your foot, making sure not to rotate your shin or thigh.

# S Arch Strengthening No. 4

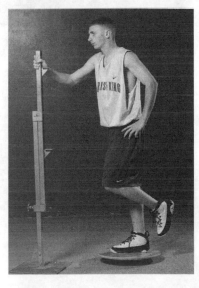

Balance on your injured foot, first on flat ground, and then on a mini trampoline or wobble board. Do 5 sets for 15 seconds.

| ARCHES | **F** = flexibility exercise<br>**S** = strengthening exercise |
| --- | --- |

# Ankle Pumps

Perform ankle pumps, keeping your foot elevated.
Repeat 50 times.

Perform a calf stretch for 15 seconds and repeat 3
to 5 times.

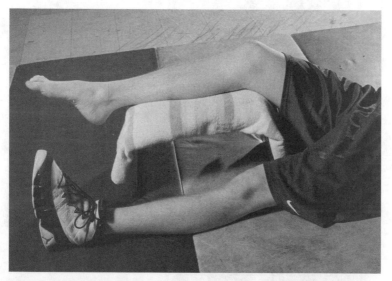

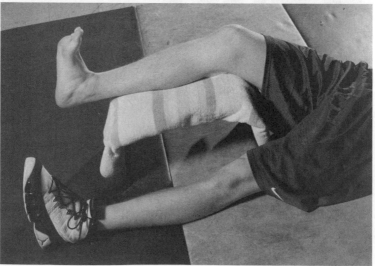

**ANKLES**

**F** = flexibility exercise
**S** = strengthening exercise

# Dorsi Flexion

Place a therapy band on the top of your foot and pull back. Do 3 sets of 15 repetitions, making sure you do not bend your knee.

**ANKLES**

F = flexibility exercise
S = strengthening exercise

# Eversion

Turn your foot outward, against the resistance of the therapy band, moving only your foot, not your shin or thigh. Repeat for 3 sets of 15 repetitions.

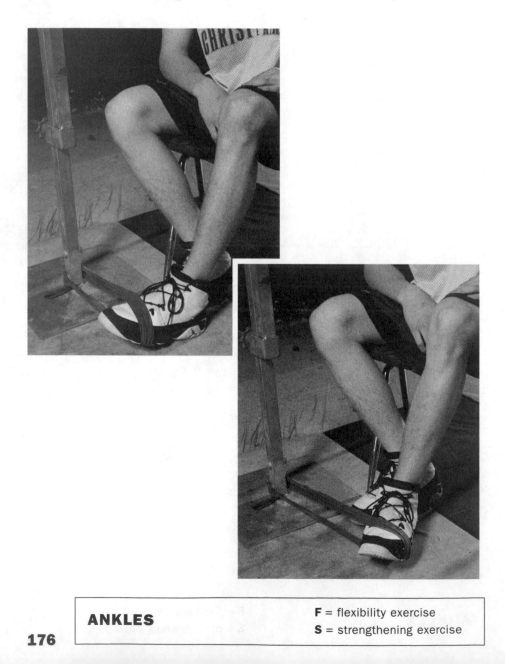

**ANKLES**

**F** = flexibility exercise
**S** = strengthening exercise

# Inversion

Turn your foot inward, against the resistance of the therapy band, moving only your foot, not your shin or thigh. Repeat for 3 sets of 15 repetitions.

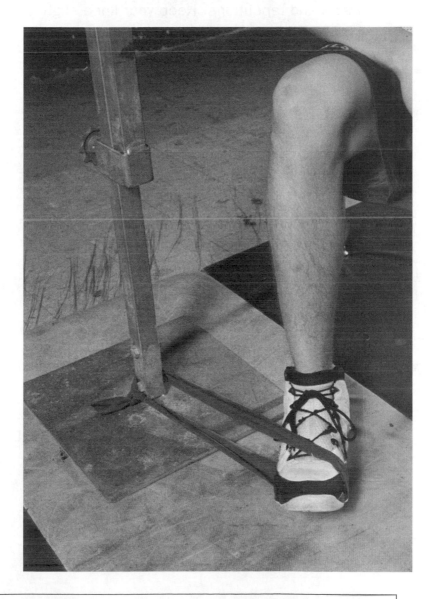

**ANKLES**

**F** = flexibility exercise
**S** = strengthening exercise

**177**

# Plantar Flexion

Hold the therapy band and push your foot down for 3 sets of 15 repetitions. As your strength increases, you can advance to heel raises for the same amount of sets and repetitions. Keep your knee slightly bent in both of these exercises.

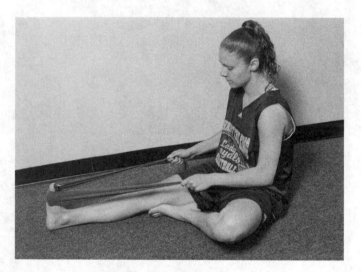

# Balance

Balance on your injured foot, first on flat ground, and then on a mini trampoline or wobble board. Do 5 sets of 15 repetitions.

| ANKLES | **F** = flexibility exercise<br>**S** = strengthening exercise |
| --- | --- |

# F Hamstring Flexibility

Sitting on the floor keep your leg slightly bent or straight, depending on what is recommended by a medical specialist. A rolled towel can be placed behind your knee to help maintain slight flexion. The foot of the leg being stretched should be facing up, not rotated in or out. The leg not being stretched should be bent with your foot on the inner thigh of your other leg. Bend toward your knee from the waist as far as you can without feeling pain. Hold the position for 15 seconds and repeat 3 to 5 times.

| | |
|---|---|
| **HAMSTRINGS, QUADS & HIPS** | **F** = flexibility exercise<br>**S** = strengthening exercise |

# Thigh Flex

If you have a knee injury this exercise may be difficult and you should start with thigh stretches as
outlined in the chapter on flexibility.  If you find
these initial stretches  too hard, put the foot of your
injured leg on a chair or any other object that allows
enough knee flexion to elicit a stretching sensation
in your thigh. Hold the position for 15 seconds and
repeat 3 to 5 times.

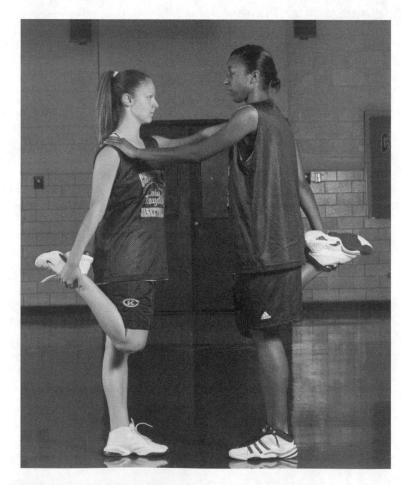

**HAMSTRINGS, QUADS
& HIPS**

**F** = flexibility exercise
**S** = strengthening exercise

# Hip Flex No. 1

The inside of your hip, or the adductors, are stretched by performing the butterfly stretch and the adductor stretches described in the Flexibility Chapter. For the butterfly stretch, sit on the floor with your knees bent and the soles of your feet touching each other. Bring your heels close to your body, keep your back straight, and slowly push your knees to the floor as you lean forward. Hold the position for 15 seconds and repeat 3 to 5 times.

# Hip Flex No. 2

Stretch the outside of your hip by crossing one leg behind the other and leaning to the side opposite your back foot. Hold the position for 15 seconds and repeat 3 to 5 times.

## Warning

Before progressing to the stregthening exercises of this section, make sure you have no pain and your health care specialist permits it. Initally, you may only be able to perform the first two exercises, which permit strength development while minimizing stress to the joint. These are referred to as isometric exercises.

# Quad Sets

Place a rolled towel behind your knee, bend your foot back, and tighten your quadriceps. Make sure you do not hyperextend your knee and that you do not feel pain. Hold the contraction for 6 seconds and repeat 50 times.

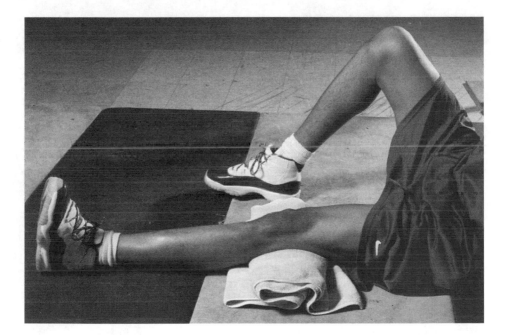

**HAMSTRINGS, QUADS & HIPS**

**F** = flexibility exercise
**S** = strengthening exercise

# Hamstring Sets

Bend your knee to about a 45 degree angle and place your heel on the floor. Attempt to pull back your foot, making sure not to move your leg, but only tighten your hamstrings. Hold the contraction for 6 seconds and repeat 50 times.

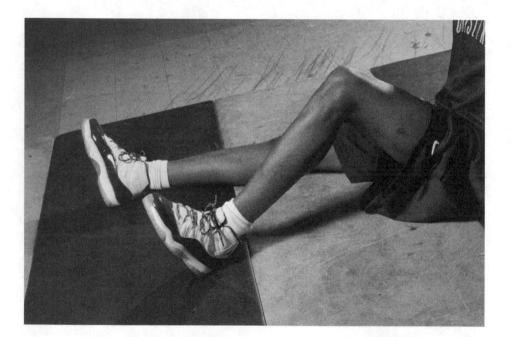

**HAMSTRINGS, QUADS & HIPS**

F = flexibility exercise
S = strengthening exercise

#  Straight Leg Raises

Keeping your leg straight, move through the following four ranges of motion. Although I would not recommend using a weight initially, over time weight may be applied directly above or below the knee joint.

# S Hip Flexion

While sitting, lift your leg about 10 to 12 inches off the floor, keeping your foot bent back and your knee straight, but not hyperextended. Do 3 sets of 15 repetitions.

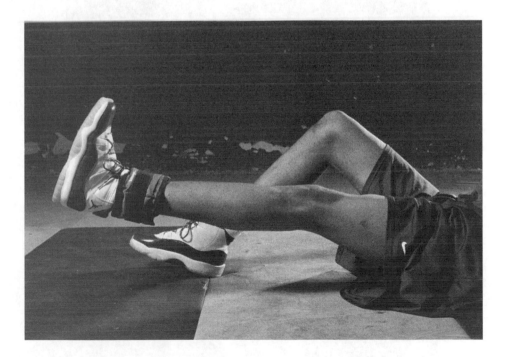

| HAMSTRINGS, QUADS & HIPS | F = flexibility exercise<br>S = strengthening exercise |
| --- | --- |

# Hip Extension

Lie on your stomach with a rolled towel or pillow beneath your hips. Lift your leg 10 to 12 inches off the floor. Do 3 sets of 15 repetitions.

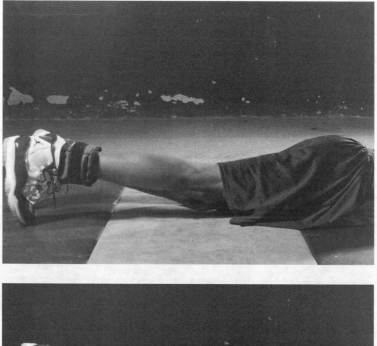

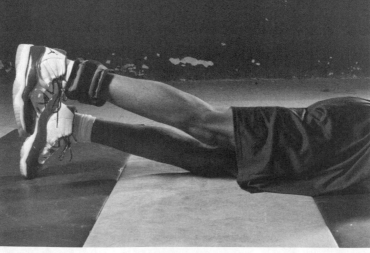

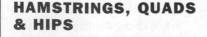

**HAMSTRINGS, QUADS & HIPS**

**F** = flexibility exercise
**S** = strengthening exercise

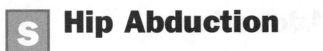

# Hip Abduction

Lie on the opposite side from the leg that is being exercised. Lift your leg about 10 to 12 inches off the floor for 3 sets of 15 repetitions.

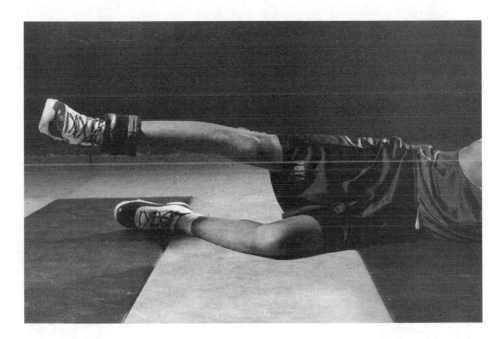

# S Hip Adduction

Lie on the same side of your body as the leg being exercised. Cross your top leg over the front of your bottom leg, placing your foot in front of your knee. Lift your bottom leg 10 to 12 inches off the floor for 3 sets of 15 repetitions.

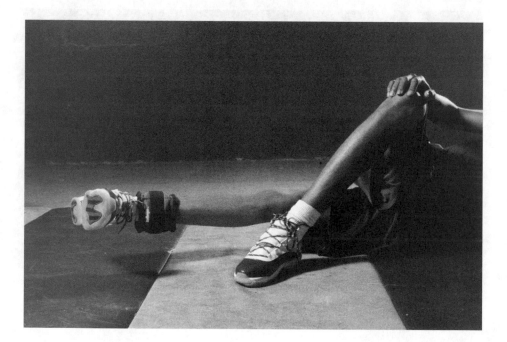

**HAMSTRINGS, QUADS & HIPS**

**F** = flexibility exercise
**S** = strengthening exercise

# **S** Terminal Knee Extensions

Stand facing a table or anchor with a therapy band attached to your leg. Place the band behind your knee and move back to a point where your knee is partially flexed, then extend your knee, making sure not to hyperextend it. Do 3 sets of 15 repetitions.

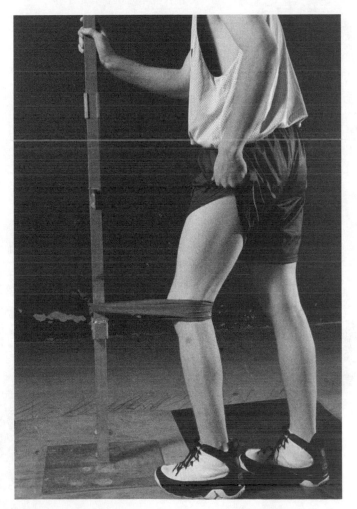

**HAMSTRINGS, QUADS & HIPS**

F = flexibility exercise
S = strengthening exercise

# Wall Squats

Lean against a wall with your feet about 18 inches in front of your body. Squat no lower than halfway down the wall and if your knees extend beyond your feet, move them further from the wall. The knees should not go beyond the feet. Complete 3 sets of 15 repetitions.

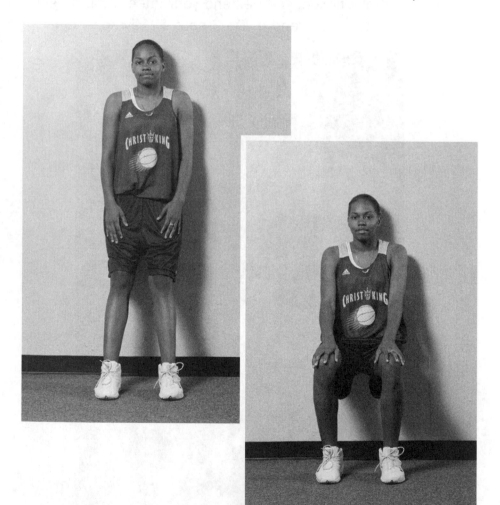

**HAMSTRINGS, QUADS & HIPS**

**F** = flexibility exercise
**S** = strengthening exercise

# Lateral Step-Ups

Step sideways on a box about 8 to 10 inches high, keeping your back straight. Do 3 sets of 15 repetitions.

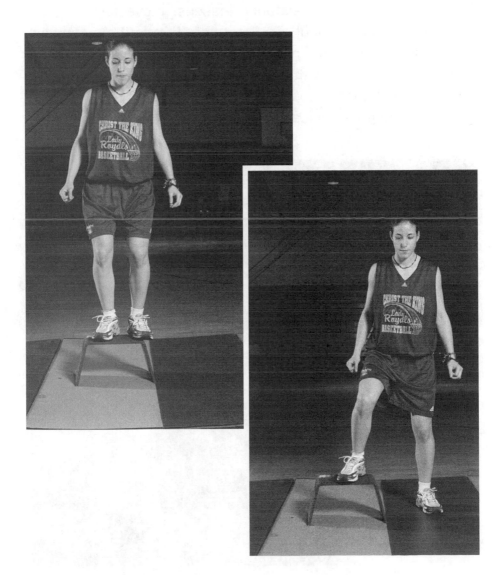

**HAMSTRINGS, QUADS & HIPS**

F = flexibility exercise
S = strengthening exercise

# **S** **Therapy Band Leg Curls**

Sit in a chair facing a table or anchor that has a therapy band attached to the leg. Place the band around your ankle with your leg relatively straight. Flex your leg to at least a 90-degree angle. As the resistance lessens, move further away from the band attachment. Do 3 sets of 15 repetitions. You will eventually be able to progress to leg curls on a machine, lunges, and squats with weights, but the current trend in sports rehabilitation is to avoid the leg extension machine until healing is complete, since it places undue stress on the knee.

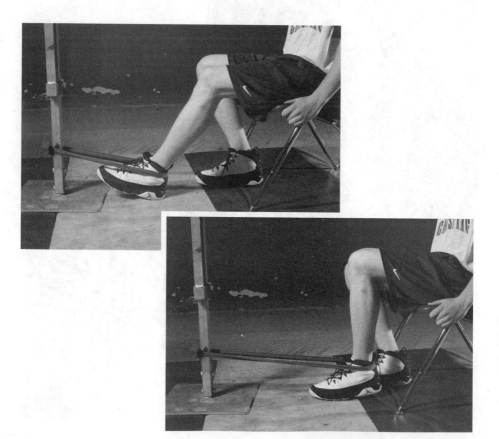

| **HAMSTRINGS, QUADS & HIPS** | **F** = flexibility exercise **S** = strengthening exercise |
|---|---|

# **F** Pelvic Tilts

Lie on your back with your knees bent and roll your pelvis back, pushing your lower back into the floor. Hold this position for 15 seconds and repeat 3 to 5 times.

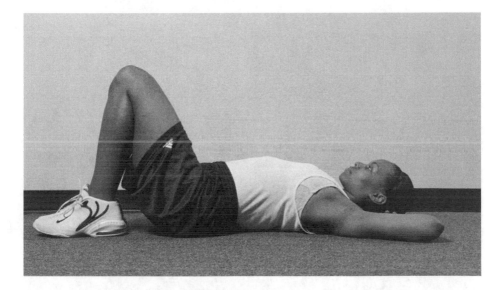

**LOWER BACK**

**F** = flexibility exercise
**S** = strengthening exercise

# Knee to Chest

Lie on your back and bring one knee up to your chest, keeping your other leg straight. Hold this position for 15 seconds and repeat 3 to 5 times, alternating legs. After the last set, bring both legs into your chest, and hold for 15 seconds, repeating 3 to 5 times.

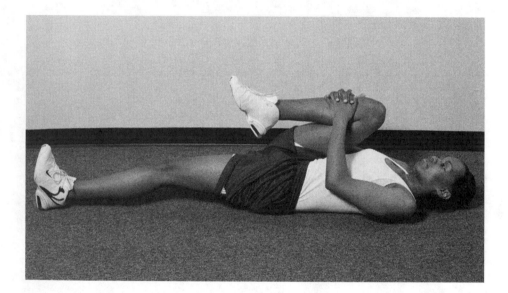

**LOWER BACK**

F = flexibility exercise
S = strengthening exercise

# Knee Tilts

Lie on your back and bend both of your legs, keeping your knees together. Tilt both of your legs to the right. Hold for 15 seconds and then tilt your legs to the left for 15 seconds. Alternate and repeat 3 to 5 times.

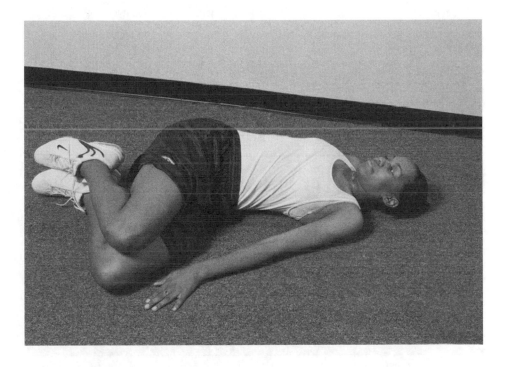

| | |
|---|---|
| **LOWER BACK** | **F** = flexibility exercise<br>**S** = strengthening exercise |

# Trunk Bends

Sit up with your knees slightly bent and your legs about shoulder width apart. Grab your lower legs, pulling your trunk forward. Hold this position for 15 seconds and repeat 3 to 5 times.

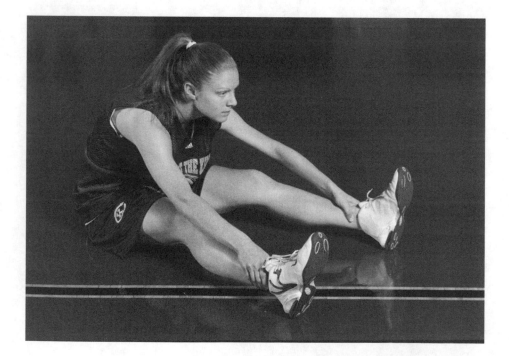

**LOWER BACK**

**F** = flexibility exercise
**S** = strengthening exercise

# Trunk Twist

Sit on the ground with one leg straight and one leg bent and slowly twist your body to the side of your bent knee.

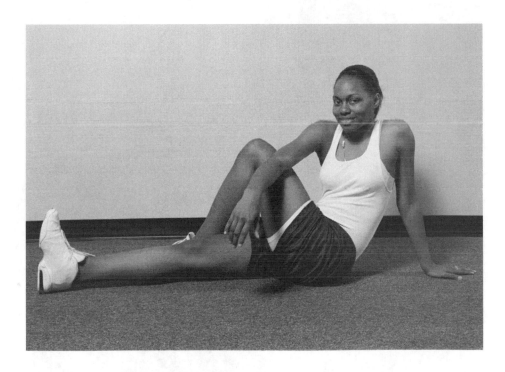

| **LOWER BACK** | **F** = flexibility exercise |
| | **S** = strengthening exercise |

# Trunk Stabilization

Sit on a therapy ball, keeping your back straight, and swing your pelvis side to side for 3 sets of 25, while maintaining your balance. After this motion, roll your pelvis forward and back for 3 sets of 25 repetitions.

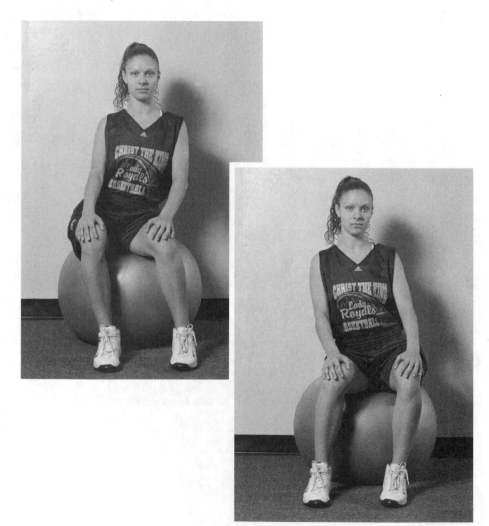

**LOWER BACK**

**F** = flexibility exercise
**S** = strengthening exercise

# Tabletop

Hold yourself up in a push-up position, maintaining a straight back. Hold this for 15 to 30 seconds and repeat 3 to 5 times.

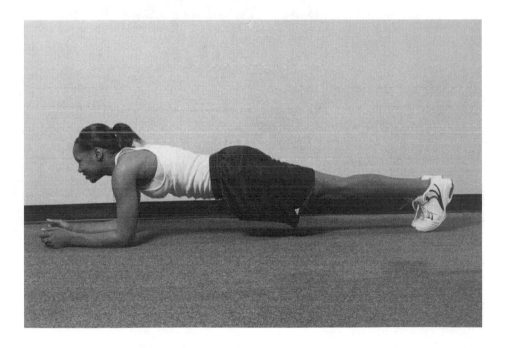

| **LOWER BACK** | **F** = flexibility exercise |
| --- | --- |
| | **S** = strengthening exercise |

# Side Bridge

Take the tabletop exercise and turn it on its side so that your weight is on your forearms and the sides of your feet. Hold your body up, keeping your back straight and making sure that your hips are off the ground. Hold this position for 15 to 30 seconds and repeat 3 to 5 times.

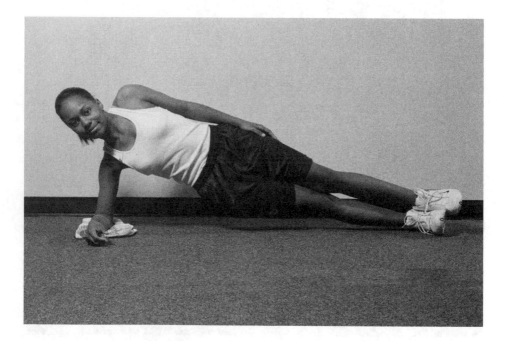

**LOWER BACK**

**F** = flexibility exercise
**S** = strengthening exercise

# Superman

Lie flat on your stomach and lift both your arms and feet off the ground, with your head facing up. Hold for 15 to 30 seconds and repeat 3 to 5 times.

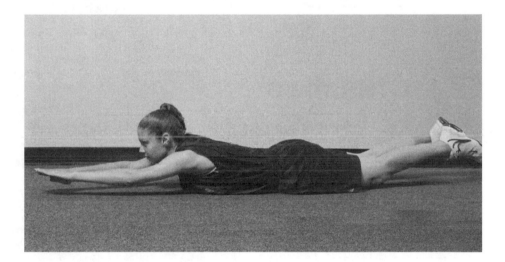

# Trunk Extensions

Lie flat on your hips on an exercise ball with your feet pressed against a wall for support and your hands behind your head. Start with your body flexed over the ball and then extend up so your trunk is even with your hips, avoiding hyperextension. Do 3 sets of 15 repetitions. You can increase the difficulty by holding the extended position for 3 to 6 seconds.

# Crunches

This exercise emphasizes the abdominal muscles. Lie flat on the ground with your knees bent, hands behind your head, and face towards the ceiling. Raise your shoulders off the floor and hold for a count of three. Do 3 to 5 sets of 15 to 30 repetitions.

# Side Bends

Hold a dumbbell in one hand and tilt your trunk to the opposite side. Alternate sides for 3 sets of 15 repetitions.

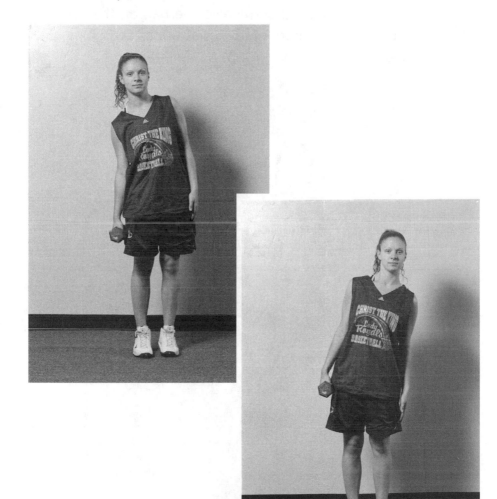

| **LOWER BACK** | **F** = flexibility exercise<br>**S** = strengthening exercise |
| --- | --- |

#  Trunk Rotations

Stand back to back with a partner, holding a weighted medicine ball parallel to your stomach. In a twisting motion, hand the ball off to your partner to one side, and then receive the ball on the opposite side. Do 3 sets of 15 repetitions, switching sides after each set of 15.

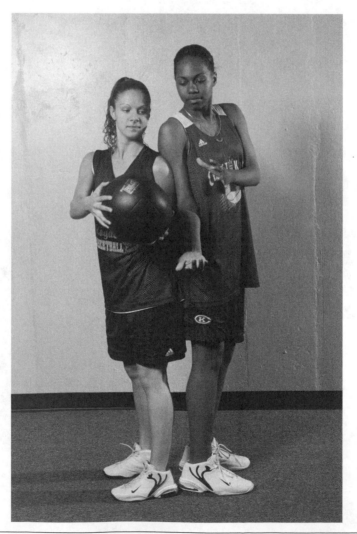

**LOWER BACK**

F = flexibility exercise
S = strengthening exercise

# F Codman Exercises

Lean over a table and slowly do 25 arm circles first clockwise then counterclockwise. Follow this with 25 forward and back arm swings. Your shoulders should stay loose, allowing gravity to provide a gentle traction effect. When you can tolerate it, a weight can be held to provide an additional stretch.

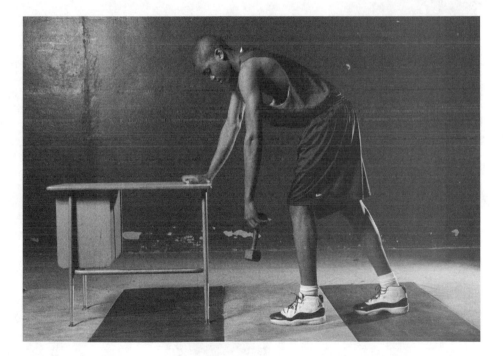

| **SHOULDERS** | **F** = flexibility exercise<br>**S** = strengthening exercise |
| --- | --- |

# Wall Walk

Stand facing a wall and slowly walk your fingers up until you feel a stretch in your shoulder. Hold for a count of 15 and repeat 3 to 5 times.

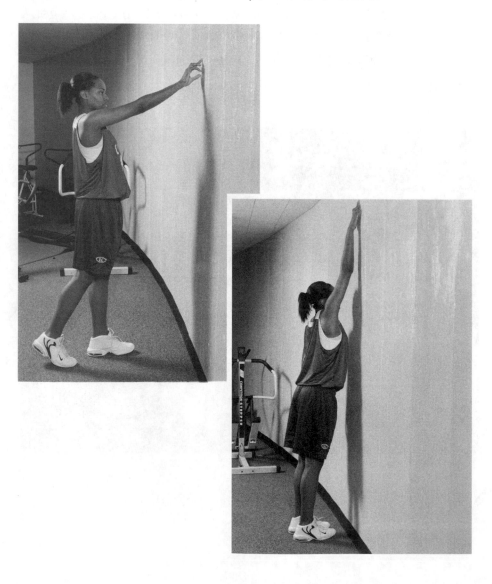

**SHOULDERS**

F = flexibility exercise
S = strengthening exercise

# Wand

Lie on your back with your knees bent. Holding a stick with both hands, lift your arms overhead until you feel a stretch. Hold this position for 15 seconds and repeat 3 to 5 times. For an additional stretch, bring your arms to a 90 degree angle from your trunk and move them to each side. Hold the position for 15 seconds and repeat 3 to 5 times.

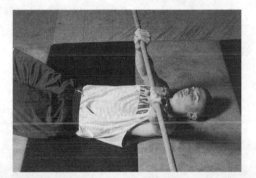

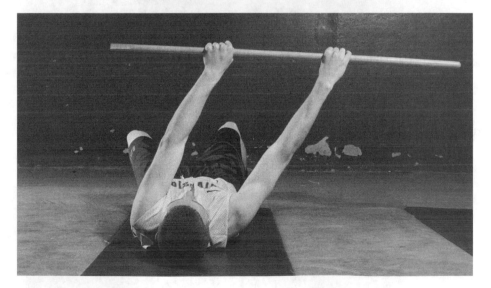

| | |
|---|---|
| **SHOULDERS** | **F** = flexibility exercise<br>**S** = strengthening exercise |

# Arm Across Chest

Bring your arm to shoulder height and pull it across your chest until you feel a stretch in the back of your shoulders. Hold this position for 15 seconds and repeat 3 to 5 times.

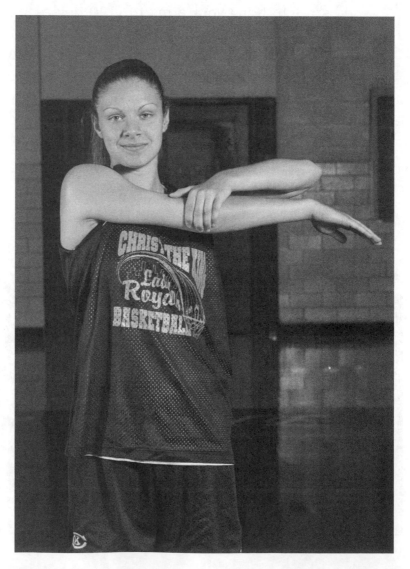

**SHOULDERS**

F = flexibility exercise
S = strengthening exercise

# Arms Behind Back

Clasp your hands behind your back and lift your arms until you feel a stretch in the chest. Hold this position for 15 seconds and repeat 3 to 5 times.

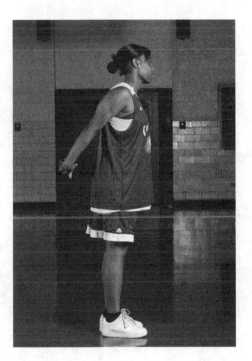

# Arm Overhead

Bend one arm overhead, placing your hand between your shoulder blades. Place your other hand on your elbow of the bent arm and slowly push down until you feel a stretch under the shoulder. Hold this position for 15 seconds and repeat 3 to 5 times.

**SHOULDERS**

**F** = flexibility exercise
**S** = strengthening exercise

#  Internal Rotation

With your elbow bent to a 90-degree angle, stand so that the side of your exercising shoulder is facing the therapy band anchor. With a hinge type motion, internally rotate your arm, but avoid pulling up or swinging your arm too far across your chest. Do 3 sets of 15 repetitions.

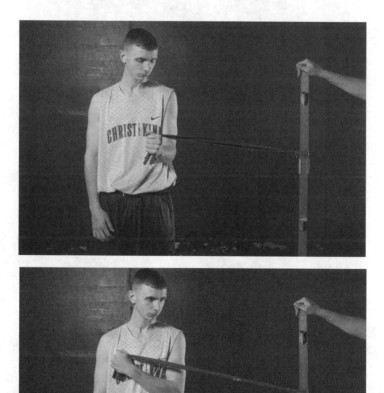

**SHOULDERS**

F = flexibility exercise
S = strengthening exercise

# S External Rotation

Stand so that the side of your shoulder that is not being exercised is facing the therapy band anchor. With your exercising arm bent to a 90 degree angle, rotate your arm out in a hinge type motion, trying not to throw your shoulder forward or lift it up. Do 3 sets of 15 repetitions.

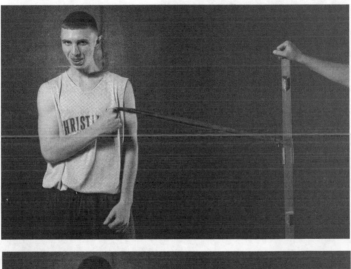

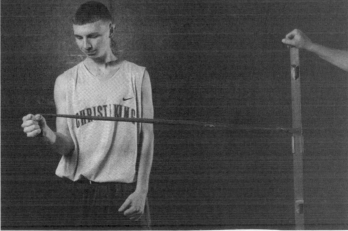

#  Lateral Raises

Either holding a dumbbell or while standing on the therapy band, lift your arm to shoulder height. Keep your elbow slightly flexed, back straight, and knees bent. Do 3 sets of 15 repetitions.

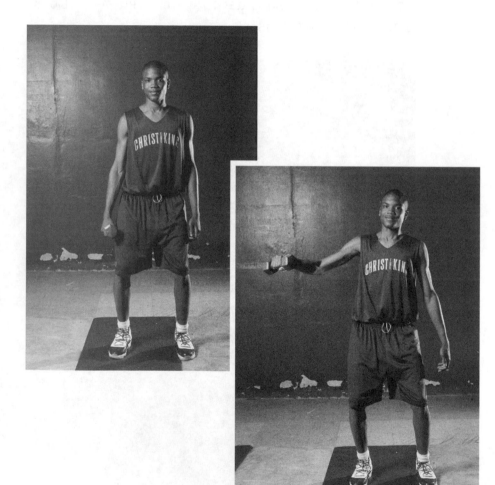

**F** = flexibility exercise
**S** = strengthening exercise

# S Forward Flexion

Holding a dumbbell or while standing on the therapy band, lift your arm in front of your body to shoulder height. Keep your back straight and your elbow and knees slightly bent. Do 3 sets of 15 repetitions.

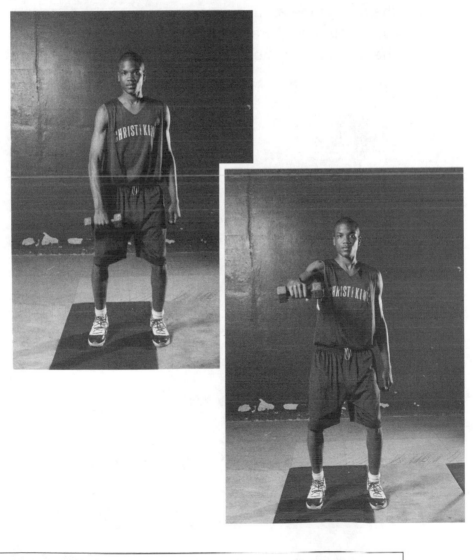

# S Rows

Using the rowing machine, keep your back straight and your knees slightly bent as you pull the bar to the middle of your chest. This can also be done as a single arm action using a dumbbell. To do this, lean over a bench, placing your knee and arm opposite to the side of the arm being exercised, on the bench. Keep your back straight and lift the weight up to the side of your chest.

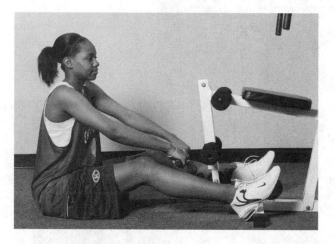

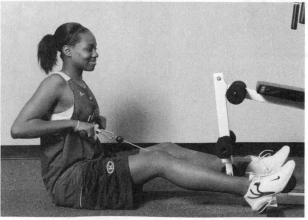

**SHOULDERS**

**F** = flexibility exercise
**S** = strengthening exercise

# Wrist Circles

Slowly rotate your wrist 25 times forward and backward, side to side, clockwise and counter clockwise.

# Finger Stretch

Slowly make a fist and then extend your fingers. Repeat 25 times.

# Flexor Stretch

With your elbow bent and fingers up, slowly extend your elbow. Hold the stretch for 15 seconds and repeat 3 to 5 times.

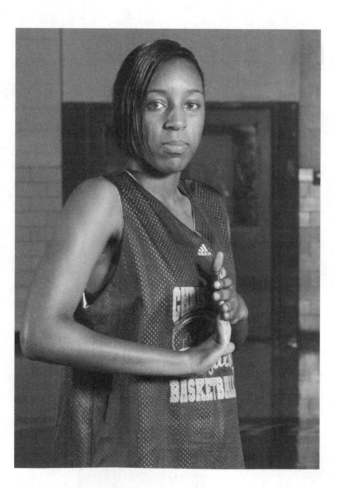

**WRISTS & HANDS**

F = flexibility exercise
S = strengthening exercise

# Extensor Stretch

With your elbow bent and fingers down, slowly extend your elbow. Hold the stretch for 15 seconds and repeat 3 to 5 times.

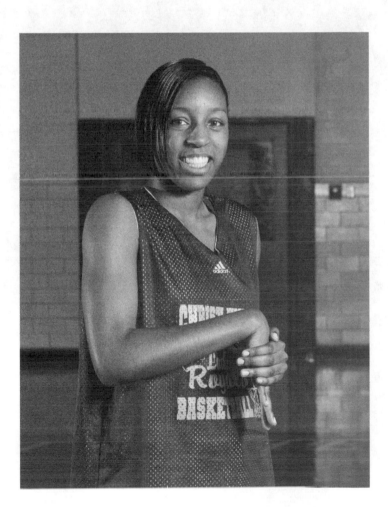

**WRISTS & HANDS**

**F** = flexibility exercise
**S** = strengthening exercise

#  Gripping

With a sponge, ball, or spring-loaded hand gripper, complete 3 sets of 15 to 25 repetitions.

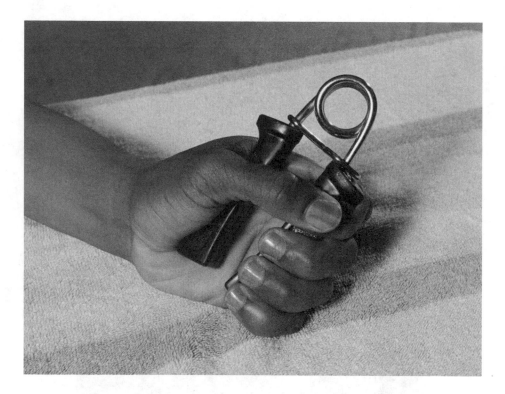

# Towel Roll

Tightly roll a small hand towel as much as it can be rolled. Repeat 10 times.

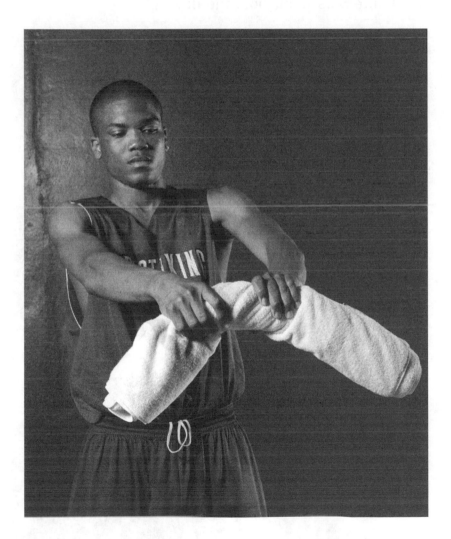

# Putty Squeeze

Play putty or therapeutic putty can be used to increase the strength of your fingers by pinching or squeezing it. This exercise can be done for 5-minute intervals throughout the day.

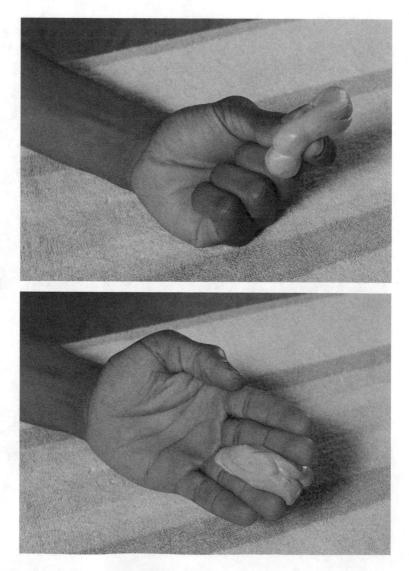

**WRISTS & HANDS**

**F** = flexibility exercise
**S** = strengthening exercise

# S Wrist Extension

Sit on a bench with the bottom of your forearms resting on your thighs. Hold a dumbbell in your hand and perform a reverse wrist curl. Do 3 sets of 15 repetitions.

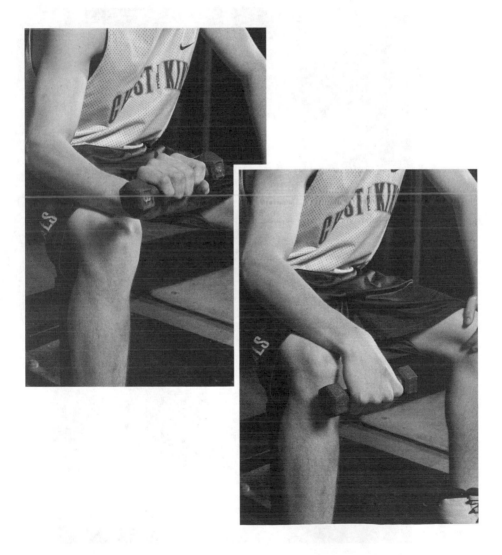

#  Wrist Flexion

Sit on a bench with the top of your forearms resting on your thighs. Hold a dumbbell in your hand and perform a wrist curl. Do 3 sets of 15 repetitions.

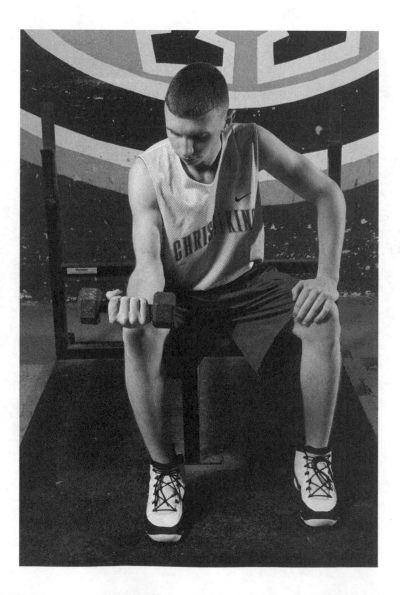

# **S** Pronation / Supination

With your forearm resting on a table, hold a hammer and rotate your hand back and forth. An ankle weight can be secured to the hammer for added resistance. Do 3 sets of 15 repetitions.

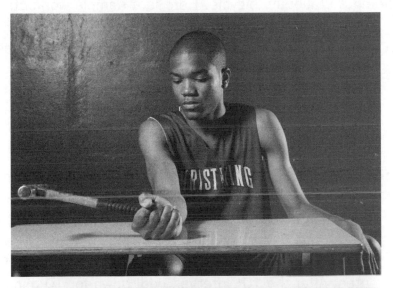

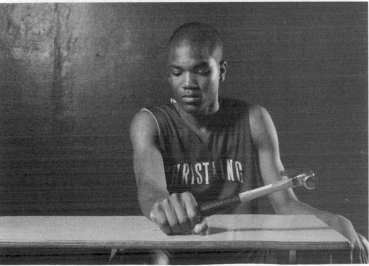

**WRISTS & HANDS**

**F** = flexibility exercise
**S** = strengthening exercise

# Conditioning Maintenance

You may have to be sidelined to allow your injury to heal. Unless your physician recommends otherwise, you can and should maintain conditioning within safe parameters. For example, recovery from a lower extremity injury can be supplemented by riding a stationary bicycle. Here is a sample workout:

- Ride the bike twice per week, 30 minutes on Tuesday and Thursday, emphasizing cardiovascular fitness.

- On Monday, Wednesday and Friday conduct an interval workout that emphasizes anaerobic conditioning.

- On Monday and Friday start riding slowly for 5 minutes, followed by ten 20-second sprints interspersed with coasting for 1 minute. After the 10th sprint, cool down for 10 minutes. On Wednesday, start riding for 5 minutes at first, followed by ten 30-second sprints, interspersed with coasting for 2 minutes. After the 10th interval, cool down for 10 minutes.

- Another option worth exploring, if the resources are available, is pool running. When you are in water waist deep you are only 50 percent of your body weight. Neck deep and you're at 10 percent of your body weight. As you might assume, this will dramatically reduce the stress and pressure on your limbs, allowing you to return to running sooner and safer. You can follow the above regimen in the pool to maintain anaerobic and aerobic fitness. Remember, use pain as a guide. If an activity causes pain, reduce the intensity or stop and seek further recommendations from a sports medicine professional.

- For upper extremity injuries such as sprained fingers or wrist, the joint may be supported with tape, splint, or brace, which allows you to run and practice ball handling skills somewhat like normal. Of course, be careful to avoid pain and always follow your physician's recommendations.

# Chapter 15
# No Shortcuts

In the quest for athletic excellence, basketball players spend immeasurable hours in the gym. For most players, this is accomplished through drills and physical conditioning, but the temptation always exists to shortcut traditional efforts through artificial means. Adolescents in particular are susceptible to peer pressure and advertising campaigns, and have the curiosity to try a substance that promises to enhance appearance and performance. Yet many young athletes do not appreciate the short and long-term risks of the substances with which they are experimenting.

Ergogenic aids are substances or practices that enhance performance. This category includes prescription medications as well as over the counter supplements.

Although the sale of these substances is a multi-billion dollar industry, the substances present short and long-term health risks and have been implicated in the death of athletes. Some high schools around the country are now following the lead of the U.S Olympic Committee, National Collegiate Athletic

Association, and the National Basketball Association in implementing drug-testing policies. Testing is intended to provide a level playing field for all athletes as well as ensure the safety of the players.

Many high school athletes are under the impression that if they buy a supplement at a nutritional store, it is safe. Yet many of the substances sold in mainstream nutrition stores are not under the jurisdiction of the Food and Drug Administration, which limits quality assurance and validation of marketing claims. In addition, many high school athletes tend to believe that if a little is good, more is better. Exceeding the manufacturer's recommended dosage, combined with the ambiguity of the actual product is a recipe for physical and emotional disaster.

Regardless of the health risks, there are also economic factors involved in investing in these products. Supplements can be very expensive, costing hundreds of dollars on "improvements" that provide similar results to a healthy diet. A healthy diet is a much cheaper and safer option.

The bottom line with any substance intended to improve performance is to check with a certified/licensed sports medicine professional before you start any regime. Also check banned substance lists provided by drug testing organizations. There is no shortage of information regarding what is safe and legal for athletes to consume.

# Amino Acids

Amino acids serve as the building blocks for proteins, which are especially important to the adolescent athlete. Protein is responsible for the building and repair of muscle tissue. The recommended daily allowance of protein is 1 gram for every kilogram (2.2 pounds) of body weight. Young competitive athletes may require higher levels of protein to satisfy muscle demands ranging from 1.2 to 1.5 grams per kilogram of body weight.

There are nine essential amino acids that can't be manufactured in the body and must be gained from food. Initially, supplements containing these nine elements were considered harmless, but recent research has discovered that side effects of taking these supplements may include dehydration, a decrease in calcium through urine, weight gain, and stress to the liver and kidneys, which filter the body of toxins. Since necessary amino acid levels can be obtained through a diet that includes the recommended levels of proteins, nutritionists see no reason for the supplements.

# Androstendione

Androstendione, or "andro," works in a similar way as anabolic steroids in that both substances promote an increase in testosterone. The difference is that andro is not sold as a prescribed substance but as an over-the-counter drug in the guise of a nutritional supplement. Sales of androstendione have dramatically increased among adolescent athletes following its connection to major league baseball player Mark Maguire.

Despite limited scientific studies, there is suspicion that use of androstedione will result in the same side effects as anabolic steroids. Because of the potential health risks and unfair advantage this substance may create over other athletes, andro is banned by organizations that test for performance-enhancing drugs. If you are in an environment that conducts drug testing, this substance will result in a positive test.

# Creatine

Short burst exercises require a fuel source known as creatine phsophate. Within the body, creatine is produced and stored as creatine phosphate. Nutritionally, it is found primarily in fish and meats. Creatine reportedly is an effective fuel source for short burst activities as well as a fatigue inhibitor.

Many magazines and marketing campaigns will imply that there are no side effects associated with creatine supplements. The research regarding its efficacy is mixed, although there are reported negative side effects including water retention, which can contribute to muscle cramping, dehydration, gastrointestinal disorders, and renal dysfunction. Sports medicine research continues to investigate the claims and side effects of this substance.

If you are considering creatine, consider that many athletes have a tendency to exceed the recommended dosage for longer periods than are safe. A commonly accepted regimen includes a loading phase of no more than 20 milligrams per day for 2 to 5 days, followed by no more than 2 grams per day.

# Herbal Supplements

High school athletes have embraced with enthusiasm many of the new "energy drinks" on store shelves. Similar to weight-loss products, these drinks and "supplements" should be approached with caution.

Many of these energy drinks contain herbal products such as Mahuang-ephedra and guarna-caffeine. Both of these are stimulants that have been known to cause side effects such as skin disorders, insomnia, hypertension, tremors, heart attacks, and strokes, and are further complicated when taken in conjunction with prescription medications.

There is no need for high school athletes to experiment with or use these products. High energy can be attained through plenty of rest and a good diet. If you're dragging and feel that you need these products for a boost, sit back, talk to a coach or athletic trainer, and see how you can safely get energized again.

# Anabolic Steroids

What are anabolic steroids? Anabolic implies the stimulation of tissue growth; associated with chemical derivatives of male sex hormone, testosterone. Testosterone is naturally produced in both men and women, though to a much greater degree in the male body. Anabolic steroids should not be confused with other classes of steroids such as those used for anti-inflammation, asthma, arthritis, and other medical conditions, all of which are administered under the close supervision of a physician.

Steroids can be taken in two ways: orally and through injection. Common brands such as Dianabal, Anavar, Winstrol, and Anadraland and Stanozolol are taken orally. Depo-testosterone, Deca-Durabolin and Primobolin are among those given through intra-muscular injection. Oral drugs have been found to be less potent, thus requiring the athlete to take higher doses to achieve the desired effect.

Research studies, medical observation and anecdotal statements from athletes continue to substantiate the health risks of these substances. Each form of administration carries its own potential risks. Injected steroids , for example, carry the risk of infection, hepatitis, AIDS, and nerve and muscle damage as a result of improper technique. Oral administration has been shown to result in an increase in serum cholesterol, which increases the risk of heart disease, heart attacks, or strokes, and impaired liver function, potentially leading to peliosis hepatitis. This form of hepatitis results in blood-filled cysts which can rupture, causing liver failure. Kidney damage is also a known side effect.

Although steroids may promote muscular growth and power, they can disrupt the normal growth of adolescent bones by prematurely closing growth areas, referred to as epiphyseal plates. More visible side effects of steroids include severe acne. Males can also experience sterility, altered libido, increased risk of prostate cancer, breast enlargement, shrunken testicles, decreased sperm count, and painful erection. Women can be especially prone to developing a male physique, deepening of the voice, developing of undesirable body hair, and menstrual irregularities.

Steroid use can also cause aggression. Many athletes take advantage of this power-boosted "psyche up" when they play, but one of the disturbing side effects of steroid use are psychological and behavioral disorders. These include episodes of moodiness, irritability, and aggressive, uncontrollable, violent behavior commonly referred to as "road rage."

Many athletes who use steroids fail to appreciate the effect disciplinary action will have on them and their teammates. In addition to the health risks, it's extremely difficult for athletes to sustain the humiliation, neglect, and anxiety associated with being banned from the sport they attempted to dominate.

# Weight-Loss Pills

Nearly 40 to 50 percent of American teenagers are overweight. This continued expansion of young America's waistline has resulted in a rush not only to the gym, but also to the store for weight-loss products. Weight-loss products accounted for $3.3 billion in sales during the year 2000. Here's another statistic: As many as 81 deaths and more than 1,000 visits to emergency rooms have been attributed to these substances.

The key substances in these weight-loss products are Mahuang-ephedra and caffeine intended to increase metabolism. Reported side effects of weight-loss pills include insomnia, irregular heart beats, increased heart rates, increased blood pressure, strokes, heart attacks, seizures, and death.

When you jump start your metabolism you will see a decrease in your weight. However the loss is not fat, but water weight. After depleting calories in the blood stream, these substances attack lean muscle mass, not fat. This is neither safe nor healthy.

The Food and Drug Administration (FDA) loosely regulates this industry. In the past, recommended doses of MaHuang-ephedra products were no more than 8mg at a time, and no more than 24 milligrams per day. The FDA later withdrew their recommendations, pending further investigation of potential side effects. Despite this, unregulated products today contain 24 milligrams per dose and their manufacturers recommend you take as much as 100 milligrams per day.

There are many hidden dangers associated with weight-loss products. Don't let yourself be deceived by claims of quick and easy weight-loss, especially with a price tag that could be your life.

The bottom line is to avoid these substances as well as any other substance that promises quick gains in performance. If you are using any of these products, stop and seek medical guidance. Don't risk your health or eligibility for the sake of hollow promises.

## Chapter 16

# The Female Player

**A**lthough women have always been part of the basketball scene, attitudes toward women's participation in basketball have only changed in the past 30 years. Before this time, many people of both genders believed that women did not possess the strength and stamina to play full court basketball. Instead, women played games of six on six where essentially half the team was on offense on one side of the court, while the others were not permitted to cross the mid-court line.

Fortunately, medical and political events finally disproved the notion that women could not safely participate in basketball on the same level as men. The passage of Title IX in the 1970s, which affords female athletes the same rights and opportunities as their male counterparts, has played a large part in the movement toward sports equality regardless of gender. Today nearly two million young women compete in basketball at the high school level. Scholarship opportunities have risen dramatically as well. The development of the WNBA, with its female role models such as Rebecca Lobo and Sheryl

Swoopes has improved attitudes as well.

Many female players and their coaches appreciate the importance of physical conditioning and its role in taking advantage of sports opportunities. Although lifting weights was initially thought to slow woman down, make them too big, or test their strength limitations, coaches now understand that if their female players are to play to their potential, as well as decrease the risk of injury, they have as much reason as men to be in the weight room.

# Program Considerations

There is no reason to keep young women out of the weight room; in fact, women benefit from the same programs for endurance, flexibility, coordination, agility, power, and speed as young men. Contrary to some reports, effective weight training can be achieved without becoming muscle bound. In fact, it has been found that female athletes can increase strength by 40 percent without increasing muscle bulk.

As with any program, the appropriate exercise prescription will be determined by the results of the pre-program fitness tests.

The female athlete does present some unique physical characteristics that should be considered when developing and monitoring a program. Young women's joints are inherently hypermobile or loose, requiring an emphasis on coordination and agility to prevent injury. Strength training may or may not provide additional stability, but is instrumental in performance and the ability for the muscular-skeletal system to sustain stress and recover from an injury.

Many adolescent female athletes have underdeveloped thigh musculature and alignment problems with the knee caps. To prevent injury, the use of the thigh extension machine should be avoided. Surprisingly, squats are better and safer because the foot remains in contact with the ground, decreasing stress to the knee. If any pain is felt, either decrease the resistance or incorporate an exercise that works the muscle group with no pain.

# Medical Concerns

All athletes fear knee ligament injuries, especially of the anterior cruciate ligament, which is a key stabilizer of the knee. There is growing concern about the high incidence of anterior cruciate ligament injuries suffered by female basketball players. In fact, a NCAA study found that women were four times more likely to sustain an injury to this ligament than male players.

Speculative causes of an anterior cruciate ligament injury include strength imbalances, inherent joint laxity, hormonal influences, smaller grooves for the ligament to pass through, and the possibility of ankle taping or bracing transmitting force to the knee.

These type of injuries can be prevented or decreased in severity by following a conditioning program to develop strength, flexibility, and coordination around the knee joint. This can be accomplished through balancing exercises and weight training with emphasis on the hamstrings. Overall conditioning can't be emphasized enough to protect the joints.

Female athletes are also more susceptible to eating disorders and the related complications than their male counterparts. This includes common eating disorders such as anorexia and bulimia as well as Female Triad Syndrome. In 1997, the American College of Sports Medicine announced the appearance of this new eating disorder, which has been identified as a progressive syndrome of disordered eating that leads to amenorrhea, the cessation of one's monthly period, and osteoporosis. This condition can result in diminished bone density as soon as the early twenties. In terms of diet, there is a difference between types of eating disorders: anorexics drastically lower caloric intake by not eating at all, bulimics binge and purge, and sufferers of female triad syndrome practice a pattern of disordered eating to decrease overall caloric intake.

Experts are having a difficult time estimating the number of female athletes stricken with this disease, but do know that between 10 and 60 percent of female athletes are suspected of having an eating disorder. The diagnosis is compounded by the fact that the symptoms of female triad syndrome have more than one cause. Factors that can affect normal menstrual cycles and estrogen production include excessive exercise, which can decrease fat stores, as well as eating disorders. Some studies put the number of female athletes with menstrual irregularities, defined as fewer than 6 to 9 periods per year, as high as 50 percent. With a decrease in estrogen dramatic enough to cause menstrual irregularities, the body will also suffer decreased bone density.

Sixty to 70 percent of female bone is developed during adolescence. If estrogen production is decreased during that time, the risk for developing osteoporosis increases dramatically. Athletes who have amenorrhea with recurrent stress fractures are especially at risk. More dramatic warning signs of an eating disorder include wearing baggy clothes, avoidance of activities where food is prevalent, red eyes from ruptured blood vessels caused by vomiting, bad dental hygiene, sore throats, anemia, dry skin, and lightheadedness.

Those suffering from Female Triad Syndrome are notorious for caloric intake with a high percentage of "junk food," and thus, a low amount of healthy nutrients. This includes calcium. Lack of calcium, combined with soda consumption, whose phosphorus content inhibits the absorption of calcium, can turn this eating disorder into osteoporosis. The recommended daily calcium intake of 1500 milligrams is necessary to maintain bone structure.

Should there be any suspicion that an athlete has Female Triad Syndrome, immediate medical evaluation is critical. Coaches and parents can help to prevent this syndrome by consistently teaching the athlete the importance of conditioning in balance with adequate nutrition and exercise as the formula to achieve real basketball potential.

# Chapter 17

# Wheelchair Basketball

Basketball transcends age, gender, even physical ability. In fact, today more than 3000 American athletes compete in local, national, and international wheelchair basketball events. Many of the teams are supported by NBA teams.

The history of wheelchair basketball goes back to the end of World War II, when returning veterans who were either paralyzed or had sustained a leg amputation were given the opportunity to play adapted sports as a way to constructively channel energy and emotional strain. It didn't take long for the game to spread throughout the United States, where wheelchair athletes from various backgrounds began to enjoy the game.

To play organized wheelchair basketball today, a player must meet certain eligiblity requirements set forth by the National Wheelchair Basketball Association: He or she must have an irreversible lower extremity disability, such as paralysis, amputation, radiological evidence of limb shortening, partial or full ankylosis or joint replacement, which consistently interferes with functional mobility.

Unlike a standard wheelchair or those used in road races, the basketball chair has five wheels and works on a low-gear ratio, which allows for quickness and agility. There are two front casters, two larger side wheels, and a fifth wheel in the back for stability and quickness. The chairs are capable of multidirectional changes and allows the athlete to jump, tilt, spin, and lean back on the rear wheel.

# Principles of Wheelchair Basketball Conditioning

Like able-bodied athletes, the wheelchair athlete must work on all elements of training. The general applications and principles are similar to those described elsewhere in this book. Those elements include:

**FLEXIBILITY.** Emphasize upper body and trunk flexibility exercises.

**ENDURANCE.** If not using the wheelchair, upper body ergometers (cycles) can be used.

**COORDINATION.** Drills that enhance the coordination required to play are included in this chapter.

**STRENGTH / POWER.** Many of the following exercises make use of the same upper body and trunk exercises described in the Strength chapter. However, it's recommended that the athlete not perform them in the wheelchair because of a lack of stability. Instead, perform those exercises on a weight bench, using spotters or other assistance.

Additional emphasis needs to be placed on the rotator cuff muscles.

Hand strengthening with hand grips or ball squeezes are important for ball control and wheel grip/mobility.

The weight program can be complemented with dips, push-ups, and pull-ups.

The upper body exercises in the Power chapter can be used when appropriate.

## Wheelchair Drill Technique

The following program was designed by the staff at the University of Illinois and the Urbana-Champaign Wheelchair Basketball Team. It is one of the world's preeminent wheelchair athlete training programs.

This workout and each of the individual skills can be modified to meet the athlete's individual needs. In addition, each of the skills can be used to teach proper technique and for conditioning purposes. It's important to progressively increase the intensity of these exercises to further enhance the training effect. It's recommended that the Power Start and Stop and a variety of half-court drills be included in each workout.

As always, be sure to warm up and stretch before the workout and cool down and stretch afterward. Finally, follow the rest and recovery intervals.

# Power Start and Stop

## Purpose

To develop the first two pushes needed for picking and defense

## Focus Points

- Hand speed
- An explosive first push
- Complete stop
- Speed of trunk movement
- Speed of recovery to pushing position

For this drill, two athletes are paired. Both individuals are in wheelchairs. One partner lines up on the baseline of the court, facing the opposite baseline. The second partner holds on to the back of the first person's wheelchair. The lead player begins by taking 2 pushes at maximum power and then immediately comes to a complete stop as quickly as he or she can. The sequence is repeated until both players reach the far baseline. The player in the back chair holds onto the front wheelchair until they get to the far baseline. (The player in the back chair needs to be careful not to slam into the front chair.) The player in the back chair should also keep his or her arms straight to prevent contact between chairs when the first person stops. The partners switch when they reach the far baseline and then repeat the exercise coming back.

## Advanced Level

- Increase the size of the person being towed.
- Increase the number of people being towed.

# Half-Court Tow

## Purpose

To develop the 10-push sequence needed in offensive and defensive transition

## Focus Points

- Get to top speed as quickly as possible.
- Maintain high hand speed.
- Push all the way through to the end of the court.
- Stop sharply at the end of the court.

For this drill, two athletes are paired. Their chairs are lined up on one baseline facing the opposite baseline. One partner moves in front of the other, with the player in the rear chair holding onto the back of the first person's wheelchair.

The lead player pushes toward half-court as quickly as possible, towing the player in the rear chair behind. At half-court, the person being towed lets go, but both partners continue to push hard to the opposite baseline. When they reach the opposite baseline, they turn around, switch positions, and repeat the drill.

## Advanced Level

- Increase the size of the person being towed.
- Increase the number of people being towed.

# Forward Partner Pulls

## Purpose
To develop overall pushing ability

## Focus Points
- Maintain a high rate of speed

For this drill, two athletes are paired. Both individuals are in wheelchairs. Both are at one baseline facing the opposite baseline. One chair is in front of the other, with the back partner holding onto the chair in front.

The player in the lead chair begins to circle the court as quickly as possible while towing the person behind. Once 1 lap is completed, the partners switch positions and repeat.

## Advanced Level
- Increase the amount of weight towed.
- Increase the number of people being towed.

# Backward Partner Pulls

## Purpose
To develop overall pushing ability and maintain muscular train-ing balance

## Focus Points
- Maintain a high rate of speed

This drill is executed in the same manner as Forward Partner Pulls on the previous page, but in this case, the back partner moves backward, pulling the front chair along. Once 1 lap is completed, partners change positions.

## Advanced Level
- Increase the amount of weight towed.
- Increase the number of people being towed.

# Clovers

## Purpose
To develop motor learning patterns and the power in the movement needed in picking and jump-and-recover defense

## Focus Points
- Explode into the turn with either a push or a pull.
- Stop sharply and go right into the next turn.
- Turns should be 1 push in length.

This drill is executed individually. Mark four spots on the floor in a square shape. The square should be approximately 6 feet x 6 feet. Mark the center of the square with a spot. Begin at one corner, and move in an arc to the next corner to the right. As you arc, make sure that the outside rear wheel of the wheelchair rolls over the center mark of the square (see diagram). Once you reach the opposite corner, pull yourself backward to the corner immediately to your left. Continue around the square in the same way, making sure that your outside wheel passes through the center point of the square each time and switching from moving forward to moving backward. Continue for the time desired, and then switch directions.

## Advanced Level
- Make the clover smaller.
- Change directions during the station.

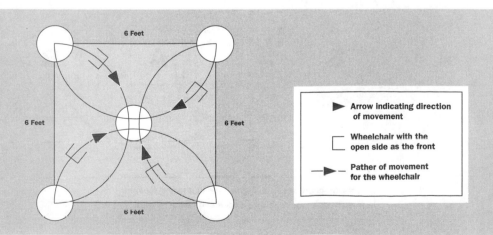

245

# U-Turns

## Purpose

To develop wheelchair control and the spatial awareness needed in picking and jump-and-recover defense

## Focus Points

- Focus on the rear wheel position and not hitting the rear wheels.
- Quick pivot
- Explode out of the pivot and into the stop
- Maintain speed

This drill is done individually. Place an empty chair or wheelchair on the baseline of the court. Begin with your wheelchair on the right side of the chair and facing the same direction as the empty chair. The wheelchairs should now be side by side.

Pull back, making sure to clear the empty chair, and then move forward, making an arc around the empty chair, ending on the left side of the empty chair. Repeat in the opposite direction so that you end up where you started.

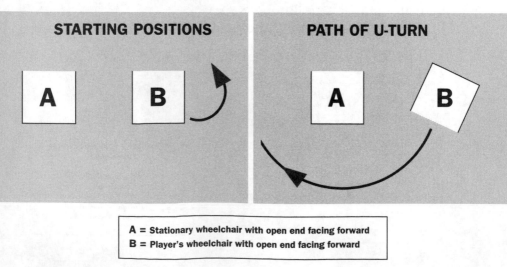

STARTING POSITIONS            PATH OF U-TURN

A       B                     A       B

A = Stationary wheelchair with open end facing forward
B = Player's wheelchair with open end facing forward

# Ups

### Purpose

To improve the individual's ability to get up once he or she has fallen, this will also indirectly enhance overall pushing ability and aggressiveness.

### Focus Points

- Get up as quickly as possible.

This drill is done individually in the wheelchair. Tip yourself and your chair over so that you're on the floor. Once there, get yourself back up into the chair as quickly as you can, using any method that works.

Repeat this as quickly as you can, seeing how many times you can complete this maneuver in the allotted time. A spotter may be necessary to ensure a controlled fall as well as assist getting up.

### Advanced Level

- Set a goal for completing a particular number of reps during a set period of time.

# Hops

## Purpose

To teach transfer of momentum and lateral movement skills

## Focus Points

- Quick weight transfer

This drill is done individually in a wheelchair. While strapped in the wheelchair, the individual quickly hops both rear wheels and preferably all four wheels off the floor at the same time. The emphasis should be placed on distance moved laterally and height.

The individual should perform this maneuver at a developmentally appropriate level, progressing from using two hands on both rear wheels to hopping with no hands on the wheels.

## Advanced Level

- Use a line to measure the distance hopped laterally.
- Move from having two hands on the wheels to no hands.
- Have the athlete hold onto a basketball while hopping.
- Jump over items.

# Tilting

## Purpose

To teach transfer of momentum and individual knowledge of the person's center of gravity in different planes

## Focus Points

- Shoulder even with the axle and the point of contact on the floor.
- Keep the weight back.
- Hold the weight over the point of contact.
- Keep your head up.
- Keep your hands over the axle.

This drill is done individually in a wheelchair. This is best performed while strapped into the wheelchair. The individual tilts his or her wheelchair sideways onto two wheels and attempts to hold his or her balance on the two wheels for as long as possible. The individual should perform this maneuver at a developmentally appropriate level, progressing from tilting with two hands, one hand, and then no hands on the wheels.

This drill can be done with a ball being passed by a thrower so that the individual must tilt to catch the ball. The drill can also have the tilting person start with a ball held overhead and then tilting from that position.

## Advanced Level

- Move from using two hands to tilt to one hand and then no hands.
- Tilt while holding a ball.
- Catch passes and shoot while tilting.
- Take a wheel off the floor while tilting.

# Tiger's Grip

## Purpose

To develop grip strength, which is necessary for ball handling and wheelchair propulsion

## Focus Points

- Begin at one corner of the paper.
- Slowly crumple the paper.
- Use only the hand to crumple the paper.
- Crumple the entire paper into a small ball.

The individual takes a sheet of newspaper that is spread out flat and holds it by one corner. The individual then slowly pulls the newspaper into his or her hand, crumpling it into a small ball. Make sure to use only the fingers and thumb to crumple the paper; don't press the paper against your body or any other surface. Once the paper is completely crumpled, discard it and repeat with a new sheet of paper.

## Advanced Level

- Don't use your thumb to help crumple the paper; use only your four fingers.
- Crumple paper in both hands at the same time.

# CHAPTER 18

# SIX-MONTH TRAINING PROGRAM

The following is a sample six-month periodization program for the high school basketball player. Training days can be adjusted to meet the demands of facility availability and game schedules, but be sure to give yourself 48 hours between weight training sessions, and do not lift on the day before a game. Coordination and agility exercises can be changed as well, based on the preference of the coach or athlete. Remember, these are only recommendations, and you will need to train within your own capabilities.

# Off-Season Program

The off-season program should run from the beginning of August to the second week of September.

| MONDAY | TUESDAY | WEDNESDAY |
|---|---|---|
| **FLEXIBILITY** | **FLEXIBILITY** | **FLEXIBILITY** |
| **CARDIO-RESPIRATORY** | **CARDIO-RESPIRATORY** | **CARDIO-RESPIRATORY** |
| **STRENGTH** | **COORDINATION** | **COORDINATION** |
| 1-3 sets | Stork | Stork |
| 15 reps | Agility Ladder x 5 | Agility Ladder x 5 |
| Squat or Leg Press | Cross-Crawl Strides | Cross-Crawl Strides |
| Lunges | full court | full court |
| Leg Curls | up/back | up/back |
| Heel Raises | | |
| Bench Press | | |
| Rows | | |
| Shoulder Press | | |
| Curls | | |
| Triceps Extension | | |
| Abdominal: 3 sets of 20 to 30 reps | | |
| Back Extensions | | |

## Goal

Develop a training base with cardiovascular, respiratory, and muscular endurance exercises, increasing flexibility and coordination. Vision and mental training should be done at least 3 times per week at your convenience.

| THURSDAY | FRIDAY |
| --- | --- |
| **FLEXIBILITY** | **FLEXIBILITY** |
| **CARDIO-RESPIRATORY** | **CARDIO-RESPIRATORY** |
| **STRENGTH** | **COORDINATION** |
| 1-3 sets | Stork |
| 15 reps | Agility Ladder x 5 |
| Squat or Leg Press | Cross-Crawl Strides |
| Leg Curls | full court |
| Heel Raises | up/back |
| Bench Press | |
| Rows | |
| Shoulder Press | |
| Curls | |
| Triceps Extensions | |
| Abdominal: 3 sets of 20 to 30 reps | |
| Back Extensions | |

# Pre-Season Phase I

The pre-season phase I runs from the middle of September to second week of October.

| MONDAY | TUESDAY | WEDNESDAY |
|---|---|---|
| FLEXIBILITY | FLEXIBILITY | FLEXIBILITY |
| FORM DRILLS | FORM DRILLS | FORM DRILLS |
| COORDINATION | COORDINATION | COORDINATION |
| Stork | Dot Board 30 sec. x 3 | Run/Shuffle x 3 |
| Carioca | Shuffle Pivot x 3 | Agility Ladder x 5 |
| full court | Zigzag Shuffle x 3 | |
| up/back | | |
| SPEED | SPEED | SPEED |
| Full Court Strides x 5 | Full-Court Shuttle x 3 | 1/2-Court Speed x 3 |
| 1/2 Speed | 3/4 Speed | 3/4-Court Speed x 3 |
| | | 1/2 Speed |
| STRENGTH | | |
| 3 sets x 8 reps | | |
| Squats or Leg Press | | |
| Lunges | | |
| Leg Curls | | |
| Heel Raises: | | |
|   3 sets x 15 reps | | |
| Bench Press | | |
| Rows | | |
| Shoulder Press | | |
| Curls | | |
| Triceps Extensions | | |
| Abdominal: 3 sets x | | |
|   20 to 30 reps | | |
| Back Extensions | | |
|   3 sets x 15 reps | | |
| Wrist Curls | | |

## Goals

Develop strength and speed.

| THURSDAY | FRIDAY |
|---|---|
| **FLEXIBILITY** | **FLEXIBILITY** |
| **FORM DRILLS** | **FORM DRILLS** |
| **COORDINATION** | **COORDINATION** |
| Stork | Stork |
| Agility Ladder x 5 | Dot Board |
| | 30 sec. x 3 |
| **SPEED** | **SPEED** |
| Full-Court Strides  x 5 | Full-Court Shuttle x 5 |
| | 1/2 Speed |
| **STRENGTH** | |
| 3 sets x 8 reps | |
| Squats or Leg Press | |
| Lunges | |
| Leg Curls | |
| Heel Raises: | |
| 3 sets x 15 reps. | |
| Bench Press | |
| Rows | |
| Shoulder Press | |
| Curls | |
| Triceps Extensions | |
| Abdominal: 3 sets x | |
| 20-30 reps | |
| Back Extensions: | |
| 3 sets x 15 reps. | |
| Wrist Curls | |

# Pre-Season Phase II

The pre-season phase II runs from the second week of October to second week of November.

| MONDAY | TUESDAY | WEDNESDAY |
|---|---|---|
| **FLEXIBILITY** | **FLEXIBILITY** | **FLEXIBILITY** |
| **FORM DRILLS** | **FORM DRILLS** | **FORM DRILLS** |
| **COORDINATION**<br>Stork<br>full court x 5<br>Shuffle Pivot | **COORDINATION**<br>Carioca<br>up/back | **COORDINATION**<br>Shuffle Pivot<br>Agility Ladder<br>Ball Balance |
| **SPEED**<br>1/2 Court x 3<br>1/2 Speed | **SPEED**<br>Full-Court Shuttle x 5<br>1/2 Speed | **SPEED**<br>1/2 Court x 5<br>3/4 Speed |
| **STRENGTH**<br>  3 sets x 6 reps<br>Squats or Leg Press<br>Leg Curls<br>Heel Raises:<br>  3 sets x 15 reps<br>Hang Cleans<br>Dead Lift<br>Bench Press<br>Rows<br>Abdominal: 3 sets x<br>  20 to 30 reps<br>Back Extensions:<br>  3 sets x 15 reps<br>Wrist Curls:<br>  3 sets x 10 reps | | |

## Goals

Further increase strength base to prepare for power training.

| THURSDAY | FRIDAY |
|---|---|
| **FLEXIBILITY** | **FLEXIBILITY** |
| **FORM DRILLS** | **FORM DRILLS** |
| **COORDINATION**<br>Stork<br>Dot Board 30 sec. x 3<br>Ball Balance | **COORDINATION**<br>Box Hop<br>Zigzag Shuffle x 3 |
| **SPEED**<br>1/2 Court x 3<br>1/2 Speed | **SPEED**<br>1/2 Court Shuttle x 5<br>3/4 Speed |
| **STRENGTH**<br>  3 sets x 6 reps<br>Squats or Leg Press<br>Leg Curls<br>Heel Raises:<br>  3 sets x 15 reps<br>Clean and Press<br>Dead Lift<br>Bench Press<br>Rows<br>Abdominal: 3 sets x<br>  20 to 30 reps<br>Back Extensions:<br>  3 sets x 15 reps<br>Wrist Curls:<br>  3 sets x 10 reps | |

# Pre-Season Phase III

The pre-season phase III runs from the second week of November to the second week in December.

| MONDAY | TUESDAY | WEDNESDAY |
|---|---|---|
| FLEXIBILITY | FLEXIBILITY | FLEXIBILITY |
| FORM DRILLS | FORM DRILLS | FORM DRILLS |
| SPEED | SPEED | SPEED |
| 3/4 Court x 3 | 1/2 Court x 3 | 3/4 Court x  3 |
| 1/2 Speed | 3/4 Speed | 1/4 Speed |
| POWER DRILLS | | |
|    see page 262 | | |
| WEIGHT TRAINING | | |
| 2 sets x 5 reps | | |
| 1 set  x 3 reps | | |
| Squats or Leg Press | | |
| Leg Curls | | |
| Heel Raises | | |
|    3 sets x 15 reps | | |
| Hang Cleans | | |
| Dead Lift | | |
| Bench Press | | |
| Rows | | |
| Abdominal: 3 sets | | |
|    x 20 to 30 reps | | |
| Back Extension: | | |
|    3 sets x 15 reps | | |
| Wrist Curls: | | |
|    3 sets x 10 reps | | |

## Goals

Power development

| THURSDAY | FRIDAY |
| --- | --- |
| **FLEXIBILITY** | **FLEXIBILITY** |
| **FORM DRILLS** | **FORM DRILLS** |
| **SPEED**<br>Court Shuttle x 5<br>3/4 Speed | **SPEED**<br>Court x 3<br>1/2 Speed |
| **POWER DRILLS**<br>  see page 262 | |
| **WEIGHT TRAINING**<br>2 sets x 3 reps<br>1 set x 3 reps<br>Squats or Leg Press<br>Leg Curls<br>Heel Raises<br>  3 sets x 15 reps<br>Clean and Press<br>Dead Lift<br>Bench Press<br>Rows<br>Abdominal: 3 sets<br>  x 20 to 30 reps<br>Back Extension:<br>  3 sets x 15 reps<br>Wrist Curls:<br>  3 sets x 10 reps | |

# In-Season Program

The in season program runs from the second week of December through the third or fourth week in February.

| MONDAY | TUESDAY | WEDNESDAY |
|---|---|---|
| **FLEXIBILITY** | **FLEXIBILITY** | **FLEXIBILITY** |
| **COORDINATION** | **COORDINATION** | **COORDINATION** |
| Stork | Dot Board<br> 30 sec. x 3 | Agility Ladder x 5 |
| Run/Shuffle | Carioca<br>x 3 | Shuffle Pivot |
| **SPEED** | **SPEED** | **SPEED** |
| Shuttle Run x 3 | 3/4 Court x 3 | Shuttle Run x 5 |
| 3/4 Speed | 1/2 Speed | 1/2 Speed |
| **STRENGTH TRAINING** | | |
| 1 to 3 sets x 15 reps | | |
| Squats or Leg Press | | |
| Leg Curls | | |
| Heel Raises | | |
| Bench Press | | |
| Rows | | |
| Shoulder Press | | |
| Curls | | |
| Triceps Extensions | | |
| Abdominal: 3 sets x<br>  20 to 30 reps | | |
| Back Extensions | | |

## Goals

Maintenance of conditioning should not be ignored during the season. Begin to taper 1 to 2 weeks prior to post-season play. This means continue with general conditioning such as flexibility, coordination, speed, but discontinue weight training.

| THURSDAY | FRIDAY |
|---|---|
| **FLEXIBILITY** | **FLEXIBILITY** |
| **COORDINATION** | **COORDINATION** |
| Stork x 5 | Box Hops |
| Zigzag Shuffle | |
|    full court | Drill x 3 |
|    up/back | |
| **SPEED** | **SPEED** |
| 3/4 Court x 3 | Shuttle x 3 |
| 3/4 Speed | 1/2 Speed |
| **STRENGTH TRAINING** | |
| Squats or Leg Press | |
| Leg Curls | |
| Heel Raises | |
| Bench Press | |
| Rows | |
| Shoulder Press | |
| Curls | |
| Triceps Extensions | |
| Abdominal: 3 sets x 20 to 30 reps | |
| Back Extensions | |

# Power Drills

| Monday | Thursday |
| --- | --- |

**1ST WEEK: 1 SET X 6 REPS**

Wall Taps
Squat Jumps
Power Bounds
Wall Push-Up Claps

**2ND WEEK: 2 SETS X 6 REPS**

Wall Taps
Squat Jumps
Power Bounds
Modified or Regular Push-Ups Claps
Medicine Ball Toss

**3RD WEEK: 3 SETS X 6 REPS**

Wall Taps
Box Hops
Repeat Forward Hops
Modified or Regular Push-Ups Claps
Medicine Ball Toss

**1ST WEEK: 1 SET X 6 REPS**

Wall Taps
Squat Jumps
Power Bounds
Wall Push-Up Claps

**2ND WEEK- 2 SETS X 6 REPS**

Wall Taps
Squat Jumps
Power Bounds
Modified or Regular Push-Ups Claps
Medicine Ball Toss

**3RD WEEK: 3 SETS X 6 REPS**

Wall Taps
Depth Jumps
Power Bounds
Modified or Regular Push-Ups Claps
Medicine Ball Toss

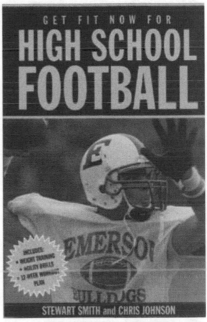

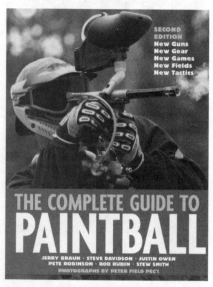